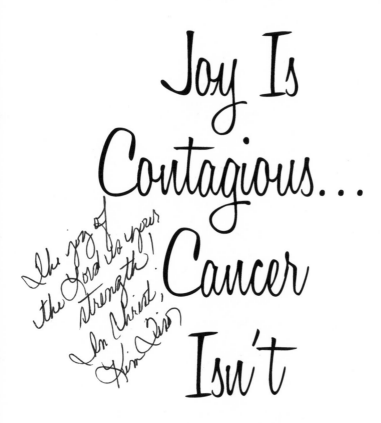

Joy Is Contagious.... Cancer Isn't

The joy of the Lord is your strength! In Christ, Kim Tisor

12 Women Share How Faith Shaped Their Breast Cancer Journey

KIM TISOR

WESTBOW
P R E S S®
A DIVISION OF THOMAS NELSON
& ZONDERVAN

This book is a work of non-fiction. Unless otherwise noted, the author
and the publisher make no explicit guarantees as to the accuracy of
the information contained in this book and in some cases, names of
people and places have been altered to protect their privacy.

WestBow Press books may be ordered through booksellers or by contacting:

WestBow Press
A Division of Thomas Nelson & Zondervan
1663 Liberty Drive
Bloomington, IN 47403
www.westbowpress.com
1 (866) 928-1240

Because of the dynamic nature of the Internet, any web addresses or
links contained in this book may have changed since publication and
may no longer be valid. The views expressed in this work are solely those
of the author and do not necessarily reflect the views of the publisher,
and the publisher hereby disclaims any responsibility for them.

Any people depicted in stock imagery provided by Thinkstock are models,
and such images are being used for illustrative purposes only.
Certain stock imagery © Thinkstock.

Print information available on the last page.

ISBN: 978-1-9736-0661-1 (sc)
ISBN: 978-1-9736-0660-4 (hc)
ISBN: 978-1-9736-0662-8 (e)

Library of Congress Control Number: 2017916971

WestBow Press rev. date: 11/17/2017

Dedication

This book is dedicated first and foremost to my family.

~ Thank you, Randy, for supporting me through what we never dreamed would become a part of our family's legacy. But we know God always has the better plan. You are a blessing to me.

~ To my children and diminutive prayer warriors Audrey, Rachael, and Race – I love you.

~ Mom, I wouldn't have wanted to face this bump in the road without you. Thank you for being my biggest cheerleader during the hardest of times.

This book is also dedicated to every woman diagnosed with breast cancer. We fight bloodless battles, yet many of us bear the scars that daily remind us that we are victors.

Lastly, to the One who sustains us each day and grants us true and everlasting victory when the war here is won, I dedicate this book to You, Lord Jesus Christ.

Contents

Dedication vii

Introduction...xi

Chapter 1   Beverly Bender..1

Chapter 2   Amanda Allcorn Graham 9

Chapter 3   Judy Anderson Greene 16

Chapter 4   Suzanne Hardister Horsley 25

Chapter 5   Joy Housley 32

Chapter 6   Darlene Sandlin Hutto 38

Chapter 7   Julie McAbee.....................................49

Chapter 8   Courtney McCollum........................58

Chapter 9   Cindy Meadows................................65

Chapter 10 Dean Norfleet...................................73

Chapter 11 Kim Tisor...82

Chapter 12 Marge Wallace 91

Acknowledgements..99

NOTES and Questions for Reflection....................103

Introduction

How would my three children respond to my impending announcement that I have cancer? I pondered that as we all sat around the dinner table talking about our day. I finally just blurted it out that I had some tests done and their results revealed that I have breast cancer. They all had heard of cancer but really didn't know what it was. I felt completely inept at determining what and how much to share in a way that wouldn't be too frightening, so I simply stated after my initial bomb drop, "Don't worry. It's not contagious," and soon changed the subject.

Cancer. Isn't. Contagious. At least that's what modern science tells us and I pray that researchers never find out differently. But something I've learned since my cancer journey began is that hope and joy are. Even during dark days, and I've had my fair share of emotional ones, we can still choose joy over dejection in the midst of our sorrow and pain.

Before we're capable of choosing life-giving joy, however, we must find its source. It doesn't come from within us. We can't manufacture it like our bodies create new blood cells (or, considering the topic, new cancer cells). We get a glimpse of how to obtain joy in the Bible's book of John, where in chapter 15, verse 11, Jesus talks about how He is the vine and we are the branches and the importance of abiding in Him. Jesus says, "These things I have spoken to you, that my joy may be in you, and that your joy may be full" (RSV). If we want to have joy, it's imperative that we stay plugged in to the source of all joy — Jesus.

It's my desire that by reading this book you'll discover that Jesus is with you, not in a passive sense, but that He's walking every step of this journey with you. He truly cares about every detail that's emerging right now in your life and He is FOR YOU!

"If God is for us, who can be against us? He who did not spare his own Son, but gave him up for us all—how will he not also, along with him, graciously give us all things?" — Romans 8:31b – 32 (NIV)

God longs to give you everything that would benefit you. That brings me to the second goal of mine with this book — that you would learn that God has surrounded you, at least within these covers, with women who understand and can uplift you. Here you'll meet women who've found joy despite battling cancer at its various stages. In some cases you'll learn of women who discovered genuine joy as a direct result of their cancer, whose days are now lived with a greater sense of purpose and meaning. Not every word of every story is as pleasurable as iced cupcakes and BOGO sales because, let's face it, that wouldn't be real life. Expect to cry a little, laugh a little, and be inspired a lot.

Three months before my cancer diagnosis I broke the very tip of my right ring finger. I'm not exactly sure how it happened, though it involved me slamming the hatch of my SUV down on it. I can attest that having joy wasn't at the forefront of my mind when that occurred and the throbbing set in. I had never broken a bone before; it was the most excruciating pain I had ever felt. As the weeks passed I waited for my nail to fall off. One day I gazed at it in amazement, the nail had discolored but was still attached, when a still, small voice whispered to me, "Your body is resilient." It was a message that would mean more to me in the coming months when my body seemingly failed me.

When I discovered I had cancer, yes, it had invaded my body, but the worst part was that it had raided my mind. At the outset, I couldn't have a thought without it somehow being tied to cancer. You could ask me, "Kim, would you like a glass of iced tea?" and my internal, rapid-fire response was, "Certainly, because it has anti-oxidants that fight cancer." Everything became about the cancer.

But despite the battle occurring between my ears, I couldn't escape the truth that our bodies are fearfully and wonderfully made…resilient. Scripture tells us that and I believe it. I knew healing would take place and that my mind, at least, would return to some semblance of normal and that I would find true joy again; I just didn't know when. I have this same hope for you. If you've been diagnosed with cancer, I promise the day is coming that you won't think about cancer with every breath that you take and that your joy, if it's missing, will be restored.

I encourage you to follow the instructions from one of my favorite verses:

"Finally, brothers and sisters, whatever is true, whatever is noble, whatever is right, whatever is pure, whatever is lovely, whatever is admirable — if anything is excellent or praiseworthy — think about such things." — Philippians 4:8 (NIV)

Choose to fill your mind with good thoughts. Praiseworthy thoughts. This book will help you do just that.

So you will know, none of us featured in this book are professional writers or claim to be. I'm not even sure if any of us are good at penning and sending thank you notes. But what all 12 contributors have in common is we've all been diagnosed with breast cancer and we all love Jesus. We also have a sincere desire to encourage others with our individual stories. Thankfully, you don't have to be a *New York Times* bestselling author to come alongside another to share your personal, heartfelt, joy-filled journey.

On behalf of each woman featured in these pages, thank you for giving us this opportunity to speak into your life when life has gotten a little harder and your heart a little heavier. We hope to lift you up and to remind you that joy is within reach and once you find it again…it's contagious!

May these stories fill you with comfort, hope, joy, peace, and every good and perfect gift that comes from God and through the hands and hearts of His people.

Sincerely,
Kim Tisor

Chapter 1

Beverly Bender

"For He spoke, and it was done; He commanded,
and it stood fast." — Psalm 33:9 (NASB)

One evening in 1986, I crossed my arms while watching
TV and to my horror discovered a breast lump. Like any
woman, my heart was struck with fear. I called my doctor's office
the next morning and made an appointment. A few days later
during my quiet time the Lord pressed a verse upon me, Psalm
81:6-7a: "I relieved [your] shoulder, [your] hands were freed from
the basket. You called in trouble and I rescued you" (NASB). I
knew the Lord had spoken to me and I readily accepted His word.

The doctor said I had classic symptoms of fibrocystic breast
disease, but ordered a mammogram just to be sure. I was relieved
to hear they found nothing suspicious. When I got back in the car
that day, I laid my head on the steering wheel and thanked God
for keeping His promise and relieving my shoulder of this burden.

Nine months went by and the tumor continued to grow. I was
back in the doctor's office two more times and he always referred

to the mammogram and that my symptoms were classic of having a fibrocystic breast. On the third visit in six months he finally sent me to a surgeon and a biopsy was ordered. I was really scared at this point because I knew six months had passed and the tumor had grown from lima bean to baseball size.

The Lord was right there ministering to me and I realized the more I praised Him the calmer I was. We have a choice as to what to fill our minds. I knew I would be awake during the biopsy so I made a tape of verses and praise songs to listen to during the procedure. As I was wheeled into the surgical room, the nurse took away my headset as she explained that members of the surgical team would be talking to me during the biopsy. But they didn't.

My reason for making the tape was now a dreaded reality as I stared into the faces over me. Everyone was quiet. The silence was deafening. As I laid there a still, small voice began to fill my head: "Fear not, for I am with you; be not dismayed, for I am your God; I will strengthen you, I will help you, I will uphold you with my righteous right hand" — Isaiah 41:10 (ESV). This was not a verse that was on my tape, but a verse I had memorized in high school as a new believer. I had not thought of it in years. The verse resonated in my head over and over. As the tissue sample was sent to the lab, it was as if the words filled the entire room... louder and louder.

The phone rang and the doctor said, "Okay," and turned to me. He said it was cancer; not the one you want to have (like I had a choice!), because it was very aggressive. He said I would need to have surgery immediately.

"Well, God can get more glory this way," were my exact words to him. Only God could have empowered me to give that response and with such conviction to the worst thing ever said to me at that time.

We checked into the hospital, and as they always do, they placed me in a wheelchair. I sat there while my husband tended to all the forms. It was a beautiful, sunny day and I noticed a new, shiny yellow Cadillac in the curved driveway outside the entrance. The urge to get up and go out to that car was almost more than I could handle. I wanted to run out, get in, and drive away. I have never felt so out of control in my life. When adversity comes, we have a choice to make. We can rebel, wallow in our misery, and be bitter, or we can choose to trust the Lord and allow Him to accomplish what He desires in our life. He can make the bitter experiences sweet. I was weak, scared, and barely able to function, but I knew my heavenly Father was with me and I was going to trust Him. I wrote out verses on paper and had them taped all over my hospital room. I believed somehow there would be a miracle because of the promise He gave me in the beginning. I was like the man who said to Jesus, "I do believe; help my unbelief!"— Mark 9:24 (NRSV).

Surgery went well. My attitude was, "take my arm, my leg, I want to live." Now we waited for the all-important lab report to know if any lymph nodes were involved. Because of the promise, God had given me back when I first discovered the lump, I was convinced the lab report would come back in my favor. I just knew that the doctors would exclaim, "It's a miracle, you had a mass as big as a baseball and no lymph nodes were involved!"

That was not the case. With 32 lymph nodes removed, 22 were cancerous. Again, I found myself thinking the Lord has this and I will cooperate with what He wants to do in my life. He literally gave me joy with a sense of adventure as to what He wanted to accomplish in me. I literally felt special and that He trusted me with this circumstance. Tarry at a promise and God will meet you there.

My spiritual gifts are faith and encouragement. I sensed that God wanted to grow my relationship with Him as my Heavenly Father and to grow the spiritual gifts He had given me. God was setting me on a path of getting to know Him like never before. My focus had been on Jesus, the cross, salvation...but now I was falling in love with my Heavenly Father. I felt special. I still had my promise and embarked on my own *faith adventure in trusting Him.*

Over the next nine months, my Heavenly Father began working in my life in many areas. Faith was one of the foremost areas. I was weak as a kitten at times and bold as a lion on other occasions. The Lord met me at my point of need at every turn.

MD Anderson Cancer Center gave me a 40% chance of surviving five years. I began nine months of chemotherapy followed by six weeks of radiation. God put me in a unique position of trusting in Him alone. I longed for someone in the medical field to encourage me — just one doctor that would say, "It's bad, but we are going to fight this and give it everything we've got!" The only thing I got from my doctor was a pat on my hand.

A well-meaning friend sent me a tape that said if we have enough faith, we will be healed. This didn't set well with me at all. It was works — what I would do. I didn't want to have to conjure up enough belief and keep a high level constantly because I knew I was weak. That would glorify me and I wanted my Almighty, Heavenly Father to be in charge! My faith was the size of a mustard seed and God's Word told me that was enough! My God is BIG and ABLE. I was going with what I knew God had told me, and like in Daniel 3:18, I was going to trust in God regardless of the outcome.

Certainly, I had times of doubts. It isn't a sin, however, to have doubts as some people may propose. Doubts just need more facts and the Lord spoke truth into my heart over and over. The opposite of faith is not doubt, but unbelief! Unbelief is disobedience and refuses to act in accordance with what God has declared.

When a person makes a promise to you, what determines if you believe him or her? Their character! God lead me to a Bible study on the names of God. Every name of God reveals facets of His character. Proverbs 18:10 says, "The name of the Lord is a strong tower; The righteous runs into it and is safe" (NASB). I began to fall in love with my Heavenly Father. He was so tender, so sweet to me.

Did you ever wish that God would just call you up on the phone and talk? During this time of treatment God did even better than that. He would speak to me in so many ways. Sometimes it would be through people, divine appointments with a speaker on the radio while in the car, songs at just the right time, encouragement in letters, phone calls, and messages from people I did not even know. But the most powerful were the Bible verses

He gave me over and over validating that first promise that He had "relieved my shoulder from the burden and rescued me."

Isaiah 51:12a — "I, even I, am He who comforts you." (NASB)

Psalm 12:6-7a — "The words of the Lord are pure words; As silver tried in a furnace on the earth, refined seven times. You, O Lord, will keep them..." (NASB)

Psalm 32:7— "You are my hiding place; You preserve me from trouble; You surround me with songs of deliverance." (NASB)

I went through nine months of chemotherapy without the harsh side effects and never having to miss a treatment.

Isaiah 46:4 — "Even to your old age I will be the same, and even to your graying years I will bear you! I have done it, and I will carry you; and I will bear you and I will deliver you." (NASB)

This promise meant a great deal to me as my children were 11, 8, and 6 years old at the time. I was careful not to declare that I would not die even though I believed with all my heart that God had delivered me. The children were surrounded with support from others initially at the time of surgery. After the surgery, the crisis seemed to have passed for them. They saw the verses posted all over the house and witnessed my trust in the Lord. We kept things positive that year of treatment. I was determined to keep their lives as normal as possible. We struck a balance of normalcy and reality best we could. The Lord has carried me and bore me through it and delivered me to my graying years. I'm now 63 years old!

Psalm 20:7 — "Some boast in chariots and some in horses, but we will boast in the name of the Lord, our God." (NASB)

Fear was my greatest weakness. The evil one wants us to be

afraid because it cripples and paralyzes us. Fear is faith's greatest enemy. I wondered if I would ever be able to go 30 minutes without thinking I was going to die. The Lord sweetly whispered in my ear that my life was in danger every time I got behind the wheel of a car. I could trust Him. There are 365 verses with "Fear not" in the Bible — one for every day of the year. First John 4:18 tells us that His perfect love casts out all fear.

Psalm 56:3 — "When I am afraid, I will put my trust in You." (NASB)

At the end of nine months of chemo, they ran a battery of tests to see if the cancer had spread. Breast cancer usually reoccurs in the brain, spine, or liver. The first scan revealed a spot on my liver. A different test was ordered with no definitive conclusion. Finally, after three days of tests a sonogram was ordered for the next morning. I was sinking fast in a pool of doubt and fear. The Lord graciously met me at my point of need with this verse… Psalm 30:5 — "Weeping may last for the night, but a shout of joy comes in the morning" (NASB). I was flooded with peace.

The next morning during the sonogram a big spot came up on the screen. The talkative technician suddenly became quiet and the only sound was the clicking as she took photos of the blob. My husband and I were numb. I asked her if the doctor would tell us what he thought after he looked at the film. She said, "No, you will have to make an appointment with your oncologist to find out the results."

After the longest 20 minutes of our lives, the doctor sauntered in casually, hands in pockets, and told us that I had a birthmark on my liver. He asked, "Now why are you in here anyway?"

HA! A birthmark! God's mark of ownership that He owned me — not cancer. We walked out of that appointment with tears of joy and thanksgiving. I looked at my watch and it was 11:45 A.M. A shout of joy came in the morning!

That was 32 years ago, and since then I have been cancer free. Every time I see a new doctor and they read my history, they are amazed. I tell them that God did it and they agree.

If the Lord was going to heal me, why didn't He do it immediately like I thought He would? If He had, I would have missed out on the richest time of my spiritual life. It was during that year of treatment that I fell in love with my Heavenly Father in a deeper way. He was my encourager and met me at every turn with words of life. Our Heavenly Father loves us with an everlasting love. He never wastes an experience; He loves me and His ways are higher than mine. And…He is closer than a phone call!

Chapter 2
Amanda Allcorn Graham

"Love bears all things, believes all things, hopes all things, endures all things." — 1 Corinthians 13:7 (ESV)

I never thought that at the age of 31, I would or could be diagnosed with breast cancer. After all, I was reasonably healthy and had three young children. When I heard those words from my surgeon, my life and the life of my family forever changed, yet for the better!

I had given birth to another son in December of 2015, 18 months almost to the day after giving birth to our oldest boy. It was a busy and tiring time! Around the end of April the following year I went for my annual checkup with the OB-GYN. Nothing was out of the ordinary then, but flash forward about six weeks later to when I detected a change. I began to feel a cluster of lumps on my left breast. I was breastfeeding at the time, so was almost certain that it was a plugged duct because my left side was always an under producer. I kept telling myself it would go away.

A few weeks passed, and it seemed as though the lumps had

grown, so I decided to call my OB-GYN so she could confirm my suspicions. It had to be a plugged duct. During my exam, the doctor's voice immediately conveyed a tone of concern. She detected some dimpling that I hadn't noticed before, which can be a sign of breast cancer. She arranged for me to have a mammogram along with an ultrasound a week later. It was July 12th.

That day I left my appointment still thinking the changes were related to breastfeeding. I went on my merry way to finish my son's birthday party preparations for that evening. That afternoon I received a call from my doctor's nurse, who told me that my mammogram and ultrasound were abnormal and that I needed to have a breast biopsy of the lumps.

The next day the surgeon performed my biopsy and remaining ever hopeful, I still felt like everything was good. That all changed two days later.

Friday, July 15, 2016, was a day that easily could have been the worst day of my life. I was at work, taking a break to pump breast milk. I was just about to start pumping when I received a call from my surgeon's office. It was the surgeon himself who called to tell me those words I never thought I would hear, "Mrs. Graham, your biopsy results came back. It is cancer."

I am a stubborn woman who rarely sheds tears, but my voice began to crack and break. I refused to let him hear me cry, so I remained strong as he discussed a few things with me. We arranged a follow-up appointment to discuss my plan of care. As soon as I hung up the phone, I fell to my knees and wept.

Then, I pulled myself together to call my husband and told him the news. He immediately left his work and came to my office. When he arrived, he just hugged me and we cried and prayed. I contacted my mom who took the news a lot worse than I did; after all I was her baby. A few minutes later, my husband and I went to inform my director of the news. She and others I had told about the lumps just knew the outcome would be something harmless and more than likely a plugged duct. She hugged me and took me to HR to get stuff rolling for the Family Medical Leave Act (FMLA), if needed.

When I told my supervisor, who is one of my best friends, of the surprising results she sent me home and said she would finish my shift that day. My husband and I took a few minutes for ourselves, and then picked up our boys from daycare.

My husband needed to do a work detail that he couldn't get out of that evening, so the boys and I went to my parents, where we stay every other weekend because of our work schedules. My husband joined us later that night. My parents were gracious enough to let me go to bed early at 6 p.m. (I work 12-hour shifts and usually awake at around 4:30 in the morning), while they watched the boys until my husband arrived.

After a restful night's sleep, I woke up the next morning with a new outlook on life. I went to work with a smile and told all my co-workers that this wasn't going to get me! I felt at peace with this situation and knew this was not going to be my death sentence.

Our preacher had preached a sermon a few months prior to this, that God allows things because He loves us. It is hard to comprehend how something as bad as cancer could translate into something being out of God's love. Yes, I was 31-years-old with an 8-year-old stepdaughter who I call my own, a 2-year-old son, and a 6-month-old baby boy. But their young ages were such a blessing! My 8-year-old could understand things when we told her, but she wasn't old enough to know the seriousness of it. My boys were too young to perceive anything was different. My faith grew by leaps and bounds from that point forward.

I elected to undergo a double mastectomy with reconstruction. My surgeon thought this was aggressive, although my plastic surgeon completely agreed. It was something I prayed about and I knew that I did not want to live my life in fear of it recurring on my right side. I was already paranoid, so I knew for my sanity it was the right thing to do.

I had my surgery on Tuesday, August 9th. Part of this surgery requires you to be injected with a radioactive, blue dye in your breast to see if there is lymph node involvement. My surgery took 7 hours to complete. When I came to in the recovery room I somewhat remember asking my husband if it was in my lymph nodes and he told me it was. Then I asked my mom, because I had completely forgot asking my husband, if it was in my lymph nodes. The answer didn't change. I was originally staged at Stage 3, but that was later downgraded to Stage 2B. I recall being a little upset that all I could eat were clear liquids. I enjoy food, what can I say?

I was discharged two days later. My parents and my in-laws helped watch the boys while I recovered at home. Our families, church family, friends, and co-workers spoiled us rotten with so many delicious meals for weeks! Didn't I just say that I enjoy food? Yes, I think I did. And, food that someone else lovingly prepares is the best kind of food there is.

When I could process things a little more, I realized exactly how God knows just what He is doing. I remember the shock and fear of finding out I was pregnant when I was only 8 months post-partum with my first-born son. I truly believe that if I hadn't gotten pregnant when I did that it would have been several years before my cancer would have been discovered and my outcome may not have been the same.

Some positive news we received was that my type of cancer is estrogen and progesterone positive and HER2-negative, which means mine is hormone driven. I started my chemotherapy treatments at the end of September. My treatment plan included 4 of the Adriamycin, a.k.a. "Red Devil," and 4 of the Taxol, with treatments being every 2 weeks. My biggest fear was losing my hair, because I was afraid my kids would be terrified. I was so wrong.

Admittedly, I didn't mind not having hair anywhere, because it made life a whole lot easier and my kids loved my bald head. I wore scarves to work and learned to accessorize. Like I told my stepdaughter when we told her the news of the cancer, I wasn't going to let this get me and I was going to make cancer look good!

As far as the side effects of the drugs, I had some bad days, especially with the Red Devil. I was fortunate enough that I was off work on the worst days following it. Once, however, my white blood cell counts were off so my treatment got delayed. Because of the way my schedule worked, when I finally received my treatment I had to work the following days with horrendous joint pain caused by the Taxol.

I continued to work through treatment, even when my white

count was virtually non-existent. I am a respiratory therapist, so sick people are my business. I just wore a mask and was extra thorough with hand hygiene. I was asked many times why I was at work and my comment was, "I have two young kids in daycare and one in school." They knew I was just as at risk at work as I would be at home, so why not keep things normal? My employer was so good to me and my supervisor was wonderful the whole time. Never once did they make things hard on me if I had to miss a day due to fever or if I had to leave early because the pain was almost too much to handle. We became like family. It was through this that I saw how blessed I was to be in such a supportive working environment.

I finished chemo in January and went for a consultation for radiation. My plastic surgeon educated me on the risk of scarring from radiation, so I was fearful of it. I prayed and I prayed for a clear answer.

When I was at my consultation, the doctor gave me that clear answer, "I am okay with you not taking radiation." I cried tears of joy as I thanked God. My journey with breast cancer was one step away from being done! All that remained was the second stage of reconstruction and the removal of my port. All of that was completed on April 27, 2017.

This journey has done so much for my faith, as well as my family's. Not once did I ever question why God chose me for this. I know I was chosen for a reason and my prayer was to bring someone to know Him and to be an example of what His love and having faith in Him can do.

As a thank you to many people that helped us, my husband and

I gave little crosses made of olive wood. One of the instances when we gave a cross that sticks with me the most involves the nurse I had the day I went home. We gave her one and immediately she was in tears and hugged me and said that she needed that. I was a blessing to someone that day. Many could take that situation and turn it into a pity party. Why do that when you are given a chance to bless people with your story?

There have been so many good things to come out of this journey and they far outweigh the bad times. I gained a new love and appreciation for my husband. He was so good to me during my treatments and during the days when I was too nauseated and tired to get out of bed. He is such a wonderful father to our children. Our families and community showed us so much love and generosity during this time.

None of this would be possible had I not given my life to God. I know, more than ever, first-hand, God is in control. No matter how awful things may get and the whole world seems to be against us, He never gives us more than we can handle and there is a purpose to all of these things. I may not be perfect and I know I can improve, but how wonderful to know that God forgives.

My favorite verse for this particular time in my life is 1 Corinthians 13:7: [Love] "Beareth all things, believeth all things, hopeth all things, endureth all things" (KJV).

Chapter 3
Judy Anderson Greene

"For I know the plans I have for you," declares the Lord, "plans to prosper you and not to harm you, plans to give you hope and a future. Then you will call on me and come and pray to me, and I will listen to you. You will seek me and find me when you seek me with all your heart." — Jeremiah 29:11-13 (NIV)

This wasn't supposed to happen to me. I mean, I'm a healthcare provider. I know to do my monthly checks. I go to my doctor. I do my yearly exams. Well, let me say "Thank God" that I do.

I found my lump while I was working. You see, I'm a physical therapist and I am daily helping people stretch and exercise to rehabilitate. It was June 30, 2015, and I had placed a patient's foot against my shoulder when I felt an uncommon pain in my left breast. I had done this movement many times over the 30 years of practicing so I knew this wasn't a typical response.

On self-exam, I found a palpable lump. I immediately contacted my OB-GYN who, after examining me, agreed I should have a diagnostic mammogram and ultrasound performed. I was quickly evaluated and it was diagnosed as a fibroadenoma. I was immediately relieved.

I went on with my daily routine of things but always in the back of my mind was that voice saying something wasn't quite right. I brushed that voice back to the back of my mind. "You did what you should," I told myself. "No one could do any more. Now move on with your life and stop this."

My husband, however, did not agree with me. Initially, he encouraged me and then he pestered me and finally he aggravated me until he made me mad. To be honest, I made the appointment with the surgeon to shut him up. You see my mother and all 3 of her sisters are and were breast cancer survivors. Three of them are two-time breast cancer survivors, but all but one of them had been diagnosed after the age of 70, so I should be good. Right?

I finally made that appointment on November 13, 2015, with breast surgeon, Dr. Pat Whitworth, at the Nashville Breast Center. Dr. Whitworth was also my mother's doctor so he knew the family history very well. He reviewed the previous test and performed an ultrasound in his office. He also felt that it was probably nothing. "But," he said, "because of your family history, I feel it would be wise to go ahead with the biopsy." On November 14, 2015, the biopsy was completed and on November 24, 2015, I returned to his office for the final verdict.

Now, I have to say, I felt really bad for the kind nurse practitioner who delivered the results to me, although I'm sure she's done it many times before to others. "You have a little cancer," she said.

What was my response? "Is that anything like being a little pregnant?"

I had to chuckle to myself at this point because cancer is cancer. It just comes in different stages. I guess it was my way of trying to accept this horrible illness. What I did know was that my life was never going to be quite the same again.

After leaving the doctor's office, I was numb. All sorts of crazy ideas kept popping into my head. Some of them were logical and others were hysterical. I cried and cried and when I thought I was done, I cried some more. I just couldn't get the tears to stop coming. I tried to smile and be brave. I tried to be tough, but on the inside my heart had dropped to my stomach and my brain couldn't make a thought process that didn't involve the word *cancer*. After several hours, I was able to rationalize some of the information I was given and start a plan of action.

Stage 1, that's doable I thought to myself. I'll finish the other test the doctor needs done. I'll have a lumpectomy and maybe a little radiation and then move as far away from all this as I can. So on December 4, 2015, I completed the breast MRI and genetics test, because not only did I have a mother and three aunts with a breast cancer diagnosis, I also had two first cousins diagnosed last year. The results came back on December 18, 2015, and surgery was scheduled for January 20, 2016.

What a way to start the year. I was 50-years-old and everything I'd ever known felt like it had all been thrown into a wind tunnel and scattered everywhere. I needed to plant myself to feel grounded. So, I did what I already knew in my heart to do; I held tight to my faith, my church, and my family.

I was not wrong; it provided me with the inner peace I needed to face the battle. On January 20, I was ready and I knew I could face this monster head on.

With surgery completed, I returned for the results of the pathology report on the tumor and the sentinel nodes in February. I knew immediately from the nurse's face it was not going to be what I wanted to hear.

"Judy, the tumor was larger than our tests showed and cancer cells were present in all 3 nodes," the nurse told me. My first response was shock, followed immediately by tears, which then followed with, I'm ashamed to say, a few words that weren't very nice and an apology to the nurse for using them.

None of this has been how we expected it to be, I was told. I would need chemotherapy and radiation, as so many women and men before me have heard.

"We got this, Judy. You can do this and I am here." Those were the first words I remember hearing from my husband, David, in the doctor's office.

It's odd what you think about as soon as you're told something like this. As unimportant as it really was to me in the complete scheme of battling for my life, all I could think of was that I was going to lose my hair, and my son, Kalleb, and his longtime girlfriend, Bennett, are getting married in June. The pictures are going to be horrible.

The hardest thing I had to do was call my children. My oldest son, David, lives in Louisville, Kentucky, and his brother, Kalleb, lives in St. Louis, Missouri, so the news had to be delivered over the phone. I placed the call with lots of tears. I got back from them exactly what I was expecting: a rock and a firm foundation.

"You got this, Mom," they said. It was the same response I got from my husband, my mother, and my siblings.

Now I had to tell my 15-year-old daughter, Brynn, who was still at school. I didn't know how to do this. If being 15 isn't hard enough, now she was going to have to watch this, too. I knew this conversation had to be done face to face. Her response? "You got this, Mom, and everything is going to be okay."

My husband and I talked quite a while about treatment and how to handle it. I knew the possible side effects. We felt it was best to receive treatment at home at E.C. Green Cancer Center and we weren't wrong. Throughout the entire treatment plan, I was treated with dignity and respect. I was never rushed through and everyone took the time to answer my questions no matter how silly they seemed.

After my first or second treatment, the thing I feared the most started. My hair began to come out rather rapidly. It just seemed like a little tangle and if I could gently brush it out everything would be just fine. But that one tangle just kept turning into more and more hair coming out. That's when I sat down and had a talk with myself face to face in the bathroom mirror.

If I had to do this, and it's going to come out, then it's going to be on my terms and not cancer's. That weekend, I called Katelyn, my hairstylist, and said, "I need you to do a favor for me."

When I showed up, she knew exactly what I wanted. I told her I wanted her to shave my hair off and she looked at me and cried. I told her she wasn't allowed to cry and I wasn't going to cry because this was my choice and not cancer's. I wasn't wrong. I feel like that was my first foothold of battling this disease on my terms. I was in control now.

Would I wear a wig or a hat? In the end, I went just the way God made me. I felt no need to cover my bald head. There are plenty of bald men and women in this world and I am not ashamed of my battle. So, I went to work bald. I shopped bald. I sang with the church praise team and choir on Sunday mornings bald. I walked down the aisle on my son's arm at his wedding bald, and I held my head up because, "I got this."

Now remember, I work in healthcare and I didn't stop working. My wonderful girls at my office, Gina and Misty, kept me positive and pushed me forward. They stepped up to the plate when I needed a little extra help and reminded me that sometimes it's ok not to be ok. It will get better.

I decided I needed to be open and honest with all my patients about my fight and my treatment. I also work with children. I didn't want anyone to be afraid of me or uncomfortable, so I took the first step and shared my story when I found it to be appropriate. Again, I found a firm rock and foundation.

I believe work helped keep me going and pushing forward. I like to help people, but personally, I don't make a very good patient. Staying home wasn't for me, and people were surprised I kept working through the chemotherapy treatments. I must have been asked a million times: "HOW?"

Truthfully, there is only one way I did it. Through my faith in Jesus Christ, and my relationship with Him, I know that nothing in this world is forever and we are not promised forever on the earth. We are, however, promised eternal life in heaven if we repent. And there it was again, a rock and a firm foundation.

It gave me inner peace to focus on fighting. I cannot possibly express to you how many people have prayed for me and reached out to me — people I've known my whole life as well as people I have never met, churches, and local businesses.

I believe, to the depths of my soul, that I could never have fought this battle the way I did without prayer. When you are a believer, then you feel the prayers being lifted up for you. It provides the calm in the storm.

"For I know the plans I have for you," declares the Lord, "plans to prosper you and not to harm you, plans to give you hope and a future. Then you will call on me and come and pray with me, and I will listen to you. You will seek me and find me when you seek me with all your heart." — Jeremiah 29:11-13 (NIV)

This is the verse that sustained me throughout this trial. God also laid the song, "Praise You in This Storm," on my heart that is sung by Casting Crowns. I have cherished it ever since I first heard my son sing it, but now during my storm, it helped keep everything in perspective.

(Chorus)
And I'll praise You in this storm
And I will lift my hands
For You are who You are
No matter where I am
And every tear I've cried
You hold in Your hand
You never left my side
And though my heart is torn

I will praise You in this storm.

Now I don't want you to get the idea that I just breezed through this. I had some nausea. I lost my hair. My white blood cell count bottomed out. I was achy and exhausted and had plenty of "chemofog" and some radiation burns, but I persevered.

And I didn't do it all alone. I could never possibly name every person who helped feed my family when I couldn't cook, lifted me up in prayer, said a positive word at just the right time, sent me a card, gave me a hug, or a swift kick when I needed it. Even the people who reached out to my family members and kept us going day by day. It is my hope that they will read this and accept my sincere thank you from here.

To my church family at First Baptist Church, Hopkinsville, Kentucky, thank you for encouraging me, praying over me and for me, and for loving me even with all my worldly flaws.

To Mom, Sue Anderson, you are the best example of strength that God could've given me so I knew how to fight. I'm sorry you had to watch my battle, but I'm glad I had you by my side. You've had enough battles to fight in this lifetime, I think.

To my employees and patients at Greene Physical Therapy Services, thank you for encouraging me and being understanding. Learning to be the patient is not an easy task.

To my beautiful children, David, Kalleb, and Brynn, thank you for grounding me and being a firm foundation that I needed during the last year. You never wavered from me or the battle. Your smiles and hugs and your patience helped sustain me every day.

And last, but definitely not least, to my husband David.

Thank you for pestering and pushing me forward to go to the doctor. You saved my life. Thank you for letting me be stubborn and hard-headed enough to push onward, and thank you for loving me unconditionally.

I have developed a new sense of what is important in this life that I may never have had without this journey. I can't say it was easy or that I want to do it again and I would never wish it upon anyone else, but it has allowed me to cherish relationships over things, to realize that each moment is a precious gift that shouldn't be wasted. Tell the people in your life you love them. Tell them every day. Forgive others unconditionally. And most importantly, remember that life is a gift, open it daily.

Chapter 4

Suzanne Hardister Horsley

"The Lord will fight for you; you need only
to be still." — Exodus 14:14 (NIV)

Allow me to introduce myself. My name is Suzanne Hardister Horsley, a breast cancer warrior and survivor. I have been blessed to be a two-time breast cancer survivor, who currently continues to fight against the monster that has changed my life and faith in so many ways. One thing that is important to understand is that cancer, of any type, is like your fingerprint. No two cancers are exactly identical. In addition, no two cancer journeys are the same. Here is my story.

Late one Sunday night, June 10, 2012, to be exact, I was channel surfing and stumbled upon a show featuring Sheryl Crow speaking about her breast cancer experience. Ms. Crow was expressing the importance of breast self-exams. I am ashamed to admit that in my life, at age 46, I had only done a handful of breast self-exams. But, that night, after seeing Sheryl Crow speak, while lying in my bed, I decided oh, why not, I'm doing one. I knew the whole technique from annual health exams. As I methodically performed the exam, I felt a strange nodule in my left breast. I thought, oh, it is nothing, so I attempted to go to sleep. After all the thoughts flooded my mind, I decided to check again to make sure it was still there. Well, it was still there all right, and now it was beginning to be painful from all the mashing and poking and prodding I had been doing.

After calling my gynecologist Dr. Madeline Hardacre's office first thing Monday morning, I set up an appointment for that Wednesday, June 12, 2012. She ordered a diagnostic mammogram and ultrasound to be done that Friday, June 15, 2012. On Monday, June 18, 2012, I received a call from Dr. Hardacre. She quickly arranged an appointment with Dr. Robert Walker, who would perform a core needle biopsy on the mass that I had discovered.

By Friday, June 22, 2012, I had become that one woman in eight to be diagnosed with breast cancer. I remember Dr. Walker never used the word "cancer" that day, but the words "bad cells" and "malignancy" stabbed like a dagger just the same. What exactly did all these histology and grade terms mean and what do I do next? Dr. Walker left the room for a few minutes. As I sat there in disbelief, my husband David held my face in his hands and said ever so calmly, "We'll fight this together."

Dr. Walker walked back into the room with a piece of paper and told me I had an appointment with a medical oncologist, Dr. Heather Shah, on Monday. My life was spiraling out of control.

Already this whole cancer thing was becoming inconvenient. My husband and I both worked full time and he could not ask off from work again on Monday. Enter in my best friend from high school, Robbye, who just happened to be a registered nurse. Robbye accompanied me to my oncology appointment with Dr. Shah and asked all the pertinent questions for me.

During this initial oncology visit, I learned that my cancer had tested positive for the HER2/neu receptor and was considered more aggressive, requiring one year of Herceptin, a targeted therapy, in addition to the standard chemotherapy treatments for breast cancer. Robbye was such a blessing that day, emotionally keeping me on track and professionally knowing what to ask. The next few weeks were a whirlwind of activity, while I prepared for round one of the fight of my life.

By July 5, 2012, a port had been implanted into my vein and I was undergoing the first of my chemotherapy treatments. It was horrible and so were the seven that followed. I quickly cut my hair extremely short and when my hair became so sparse that I looked like an alien, my husband shaved my remaining hair with his clippers, as my two youngest children watched and sobbed.

Every other Thursday, after my chemotherapy treatments, a precious friend brought food for me and my family. I learned that many people that you expect to be there to emotionally support you are often absent, but many people that you never expected would step up and fill the void.

Every afternoon I would walk to the mailbox to find cards and letters of encouragement. I would receive phone calls from people I had not talked to in years. One thing remained constant — my belief that God was in control. After eight cycles of chemotherapy, in November 2012, I had a double mastectomy. Maintenance Herceptin infusions were continued until the end of July 2013. I had finished my treatments and my scans were clear. I had won the battle. My life could get back to normal! I was elated!

I had plans, like starting a new career and having a schedule that I could totally control! This was my plan, but God's plan was different than mine. In February 2014, a sore, aching left arm caused me concern and I felt a small nodule under my left arm. I had an appointment scheduled with my surgeon, Dr. Walker, to discuss port removal. Instead, a biopsy on the lymph node was performed and on February 25, 2014, biopsy results revealed that the cancer had returned.

On March 10, 2014, all 27 axillary lymph nodes were removed and all tested malignant. I was told the returning cancer was once again HER2/neu positive and was even more aggressive than before. My disease, while technically the same, was different. The oncologist said my treatment plan would cause much more toxicity. I just knew that would not be the case with me.

With my first diagnosis, I worked on Thursday until noon and pushed myself back to work by Monday. Well, mind over matter did not work with round two. I became frustrated. The cancer fight is far from fun and far from simple. It creates complex thoughts and emotions. More aggressive cancer meant more aggressive chemotherapy. My treatments caused blood poisoning, nausea, fatigue, repeat hair loss, neuropathy, and weakened my heart to within 6% of heart failure.

In July 2014, a decision was made to remove two of the four drugs from my treatment regime that I received via infusion every three weeks. The decision was also made that I would receive two targeted therapies, Herceptin and Perjeta, for an indefinite amount of time, and if my heart would tolerate it, probably the rest of my life. In addition, I would undergo 35 radiation treatments. The truth is I never really got mad. Here is an analogy I used when asked about my cancer. You had to board a plane. It was not an option, you absolutely had to board it. If the flight attendant looked at you and said, "This plane is going to crash and you will have very serious injuries. You will have less than a 50% chance of surviving for five years," how would you spend your time? This scenario was very similar to the cards I have been dealt.

Life is short and time passes quickly. I remember a history teacher I had in high school used to respond to students who would ask her what time it was by saying, "Time will pass, will you?" No truer words have been spoken. When I was in pain or I was feeling like a pin cushion, I would take my mind to another place by thinking this is temporary. After all, that mentality got me through an unplanned natural child birth of an 8 lb., 10 oz., baby girl.

I often found myself, even as an adult, wishing days away. That is one thing an illness like cancer will stop you from doing, wishing precious days away. Every single day, whether it is a day filled with fun activities or a mundane day doing something less fun, is a day to make a difference, change for the better, bring joy to both people close to you or new acquaintances.

I have found joy in things I used to see as insignificant and trivial. My illness made me put the brakes on life and take control. In the beginning of my recurrence and the less than positive prognosis, I was not sure I would be able to ever get to the point that I could find a blessing in all of this craziness, like I did with my first diagnosis. With my first diagnosis, I was going to be that strong breast cancer survivor that I wanted to be. With the second diagnosis, it was hard to focus on being the survivor because of the fear of the unknown. But honestly, isn't life just one big unknown?

I had to make some difficult decisions to eliminate people and things from my life that put conditions on how I was supposed to feel and would not allow me to get my life in a "good place." I would encourage everyone to be proactive and not wait until you hear something that puts fear in you to get your life in a good place spiritually or emotionally. Not everyone gets the luxury of the time to be able to do that.

I love the relationships that cancer helped me foster. I love my friends, both old and new. I love all the cards I received in the mail that gave me encouragement. I love the friends that took the time out of their busy lives to bring me and my family a warm, delicious meal. I love my breast cancer support group, "The Rack Pack." This group brought so many wonderful people into my life.

I loved the time with my mother when she practically lived with me to take care of me. I am so blessed to be the recipient of her unconditional love and efforts that helped me fight so hard, even if she was the "Food Nazi!" You laugh at that, but she wouldn't allow any foods she deemed unclean to enter my family's menu or my mouth.

I love my oncologist, Dr. Shah, for her intense knowledge of my disease and her love and compassion for patients like me. I love her nurse, Melissa, who I can cry and laugh with and is never too busy to speak with me about sometimes things that may not be that important. Last, but certainly not least, I love my husband and children for their unwavering love for me, a woman who because of all her illnesses and surgeries, sometimes feels like an incomplete wife and mother.

Love every minute of life. Cherish every day and make a difference! My illness has made me want to create a great legacy.

God is good all the time, even during the struggles. Remember, we may not know God's plan, but He doesn't make mistakes. There is a reason for everything. "The Lord will fight for you; you need only to be still."— Exodus 14:14 (NIV)

Chapter 5
Joy Housley

"I can do all things through Christ which strengtheneth me."
— Philippians 4:13 (KJV)

The sound of silence...that was the first thing I remember in 1998, when my doctor told me he was sure the lump in my breast was cancer. My husband and I just looked at each other.

The 40-mile trip home seemed like 100. I didn't know what to do, who to call first. But I knew I had to call my mother, and that would be a very difficult call to make. You see, I had just lost my father to lung cancer two months prior and we were all still on that emotional roller coaster.

It all started on a Friday when I discovered the lump in my breast. I called and scheduled an appointment with my gynecologist for the following Monday. She did an ultrasound and immediately sent me over to the breast center for a mammogram. After seeing the results, she recommended that I see a surgeon. The following day we were in the surgeon's office discussing our options. One week later I was in the hospital having surgery to remove my left breast. Talk about another emotional roller coaster ride! Along with the surgery, they removed 10 lymph nodes, three of which were also cancer. I was diagnosed with Stage IIB, ductal carcinoma breast cancer.

I never asked, "Why me, Lord?" I trusted Him to take care of me.

I went through chemo and reconstruction that first year and when I reached my five-year mark with no reoccurrence, I thought I was cancer free. God still had plans for me. Life was good.

In January of 2012, my husband, Edgar, was having severe shoulder pain. Our family physician had passed away a few months prior and we had been putting off finding a new doctor. After several recommendations, I found a doctor that was taking new patients and made an appointment for him. I was impressed with our new find and decided to make an appointment for myself, since I had been having shortness of breath and a cough that wouldn't go away.

After a routine physical my doctor ordered blood work and a chest x-ray. Needless to say, we got that dreaded phone call on Valentine's Day that my blood work didn't look good and something showed up on the x-ray. He wanted me back in for further tests. After all tests were in we found out that my breast cancer had returned and spread to my lungs, my bones, and one lymph node.

This time I was terrified, as well as Edgar, my "fixer." I remember nights in bed holding each other and crying. We knew what Stage IV meant.

Once more it was all in God's hands. He brought me through it the first time, but would He do it again?

My oncologist took over and mapped out a plan that didn't involve chemotherapy this time. My cancer was affected by a protein found on the surface of my cancer cells that grows and divides quickly creating more cancer cells. We started the fight using an immune targeted therapy known as blockers, along with estrogen blocking medications, and bone strengthening injections. I'm on what I call a maintenance plan, infusions for the targeted therapy every two weeks, daily medication for the estrogen and injections for my bones once a month. I'll be on this plan for the rest of my life, as long as they continue to work.

I know that God also has a maintenance plan for me and one that will never fail. His daily infusions are what keep me going. Without Him I would have given up years ago. "My flesh and my heart faileth: but God is the strength of my heart, and my portion forever." — Psalms 73:26 (KJV).

Through all of this, I have found out that Stage IV breast cancer is not an immediate death sentence. Although there is no cure, there are treatments that can keep it at bay and hopefully prolong life. So far the worst part of treatment for me has been the infamous side effects. Each comes with their own unique blend, but the most common side effect of many is fatigue. Fatigue related to cancer is different from fatigue that healthy people feel. We cannot get relief by sleep or rest and it disrupts our lives tremendously.

I've also had to have radiation twice since my reoccurrence to relieve bone pain. And although each time it has helped with the pain, along with it comes its own side effects.

I had radiation a year ago for pain in my shoulder, neck, and jaw. Almost immediately I started having a severe sore throat and trouble swallowing. It took about 6 weeks for the throat to quit hurting, but I still couldn't swallow very well and had developed a constant cough. Back to the oncologist for more testing. After several scans and no known culprit, he sent me to a pulmonary specialist. He, in turn, sent me to the hospital for a Pulmonary Function Test.

During this test, I was given a high dose of Albuterol and upon leaving the hospital, I collapsed in the main lobby and had to be rushed to the ER. I was having trouble breathing, jerking all over, and didn't have the ability to tell anyone what was wrong. I thought I was having a heart attack. Several hours later it was confirmed that I am allergic to Albuterol.

The results from my Pulmonary Function Test turned out to be normal for a person with my diagnosis, so he sent me to an Ear, Nose, and Throat specialist. I didn't have much faith in this specialist because I was so sure that my coughing, shortness of breath, and swallowing issues were all related to my cancer.

The ENT doctor did a scope of my throat and told me exactly what was going on. It seems that the radiation had shrunk the muscles around my larynx. We went in to surgery shortly afterwards for an esophagus dilation (throat stretching), which only helped for about three days. So, it seems I'm going to have to live with this. YUK!

Even with all my issues, my life has been blessed. I have a

wonderful, supportive family and I'm grateful beyond measure for my husband Edgar. We were married a little less than three years when I received my first diagnosis. He's wiped my tears, held me, cried with me, and supported every decision I've made concerning my cancer and treatments.

I have a locket that I wear that has a picture of a young boy that stole my heart the minute he was born. He couldn't have been more precious to me than if he were my own child. Anyone who has a grandchild will know exactly what I am talking about. I couldn't bear to think about not being here to watch him grow up. I'm glad the Lord has allowed me the privilege. I have watched him grow into a bright young man. He is intelligent, clever, and very humorous. He has a good heart and is making his way to becoming a physical therapist. I opted for a plastic surgeon, but he had his mind made up.

My children have always been there for me. I'm so very proud of them and the adults they've become. Sometimes I wonder how I was so lucky. I'm thankful that the Lord has given me this extra time with them. Many people, regardless of cancer, have not been so fortunate.

I have a dear friend that lost her daughter to breast cancer just a few years ago. She left behind two young children. She was a loving wife and mother. I have often asked God why did He take a young mother with so much more left to do and not someone like me instead. I haven't received my answer yet.

Difficult times have often been referred to as storms in our lives. How do we prepare? Just because we're in a storm doesn't mean that God isn't there. Remember the disciples out in the Sea of Galilee? They were afraid even when they saw Jesus. I'll have to say that I have been terrified at times, especially while waiting on scan results. I give my worries to Him, but then I take them back. And that is not what He teaches us to do. But I know I have focused more on Him through this walk with cancer than ever before. His works have benefited me and I hope they have blessed others through me. I have found God faithful, loving, and merciful, especially through my storms. And even though I will never have this storm behind me, He calms me and grows more dear and precious to me every day.

"Feed your faith and your fears will starve to death." — Author Unknown

P.S. Remember that shoulder pain that Edgar had and we were forced to find a new doctor? They never found a reason for the pain and he never had any more trouble after that initial visit. The Lord knew how to get my attention....

Chapter 6
Darlene Sandlin Hutto

"With men this is impossible; but with God all
things are possible." — Matthew 19:26 (KJV)

I began having yearly mammograms after my mother was
diagnosed with breast cancer in 2003. Each year, like
clockwork, I was given a clean bill of health. So, it came as a
surprise when six months after my mammogram and ultrasound
in May of 2014, that there arose a cause for concern. Real concern.

It was November 2014, when I felt a sore spot at the top of
my right breast. I assumed it was from some of the exercises I was
doing at the gym. I couldn't feel anything out of the ordinary
when I performed a breast self-exam. Once we got through the
holidays and into the New Year I decided that I should go to the
doctor to have it checked out.

My gynecologist scheduled a mammogram of my right
breast. He called me later and said the radiologist saw something
suspicious, but thought it could be infection. It was not at the top
where the sore spot was and he said most of the time cancer would

not make you sore. I still don't know what caused the sore spot. I believe God put it there so I would go to the doctor. I was given an antibiotic to take for a couple of weeks and then returned for an ultrasound. The radiologist still saw something but was "iffy" on what it was. My gynecologist said he would feel better if I had a biopsy to make sure.

The spot they were seeing was at the bottom of my breast and deep inside, closer to the muscle. I had to go to the mammography center for an ultrasound guided biopsy because the spot was so small, so small that you couldn't feel it.

My whole world changed on March 5, 2015, when at the age of 49, I got the call informing me that I had breast cancer. My entire body went numb and my mind went in a million directions. My husband was at home with me that day because we had snow and he was unable to go to work.

From the very beginning, I put it in God's hands. I knew there was nothing I could do to change anything. I had to trust in God to take care of me. This is not to say that I didn't have my days when I was scared or down, because I did have those days. That's only natural. I would pray and ask God to help me and He did. God gave me a peace that no one else could have provided. Some Bible verses that became very important to me were:

"Do not be afraid or discouraged because of this vast army. For the battle is not yours, but God's." — 2 Chronicles 20:15 (NIV)

"When I am afraid, I put my trust in you." — Psalm 56:3 (NIV)

"The Lord will fight for you; you need only to be still." — Exodus 14:14 (NIV)

I met with my surgeon to discuss options for surgery and with a plastic surgeon to discuss reconstruction options. Because I had dense breast tissue, I made the decision to have a double mastectomy. I couldn't help but wonder if having dense tissue prevented my cancer from being discovered earlier.

Spring break was coming up and my plastic surgeon would be out of town for a week. He said he could do the surgery on March 16th, or after spring break. I wanted the cancer out of my body as soon as I could, so we scheduled my surgery for March 16th.

My surgeon performed the double mastectomy and my plastic surgeon put the expanders in during the 4½ hour surgery. I was in a good bit of pain afterward so I was given a pain pump with morphine. My daughter kept a very detailed notebook for me about what happened while I was in the hospital so I would have it as a keepsake. I am so thankful she did this for me!

The hospital discharged me to go home Thursday, March 19th. My plastic surgeon took two of the five drain tubes that were placed during surgery out the following day, two more the next Monday, and the last drain was taken out on Wednesday. I remember that while at home I was very sore when trying to get up and down and my chest and ribs hurt a lot! The pain was so intense that at one point I called my plastic surgeon because I thought something was wrong. He assured me that the pain was normal.

I had my post-op appointment with my surgeon on April 1st, and got my pathology report. It was Stage 3 invasive mammary carcinoma and abundant ductal carcinoma in situ, which had spread to 13 out of 16 lymph nodes. The type was Triple Negative. This news terrified me because this is a very aggressive type of breast cancer. After the initial shock of hearing my diagnosis, I realized again that there was nothing I could do, I had to trust God and He would help me get through this.

I went back to my plastic surgeon several times for him to add saline to my expanders. Each time, they became more uncomfortable because it was stretching my skin and pushing down on my ribs.

One day before I began chemo, I went to a local wig shop called Special Touch by Eunice. Eunice and all her staff are breast cancer survivors, so they were very compassionate and helpful. While I was there, Eunice gave me a copy of the poem "Attitudes" by Charles R. Swindoll. Having the right attitude, as the poem explains, is everything! Hopefully it encourages you the way it did me.

Attitudes

The longer I live, the more I realize the importance
of choosing the right attitude in life.
Attitude is more important than facts.
It is more important than your past;
more important than your education or your financial situation;
more important than your circumstances,
your successes, or your failures;
more important than what other people think or say or do.
It is more important than your appearance,
your giftedness, or your skills.

It will make or break a company. It will
cause a church to soar or sink.
It will make the difference between a
happy home or a miserable home.
You have a choice each day regarding
the attitude you will embrace.

Life is like a violin.
You can focus on the broken strings that dangle,
or you can play your life's melody on the one that remains.
You cannot change the years that have passed,
nor can you change the daily tick of the clock.
You cannot change the pace of your march toward your death.
You cannot change the decisions or reactions of other people.
And you certainly cannot change the inevitable.
Those are strings that dangle!
What you can do is play on the one string
that remains – your attitude.
I am convinced that life is 10 percent what happens to me
and 90 percent how I react to it.
The same is true for you.

As I was leaving the store, I met another customer named
Carrie. She was an older, frail looking lady who was a breast
cancer survivor. She gave me a hug and asked if she could pray
for me. Of course, I said, "Yes, I would love that!" She prayed the
sweetest prayer. I will never forget her. She was such a blessing
and inspiration to me.

God continued to put people in my life that would help me

on this journey. I believe that God uses every situation for His good. I never would have met some of the most precious ladies who are so important to me now, had I not been diagnosed with breast cancer. One breast cancer survivor contacted me via email and told me her story, which really helped me to have an idea of what to expect as I went through my surgery and treatments. She was a member of a local breast cancer support group called The Rack Pack…I love this name. She invited me to come to a meeting when I felt like it. I went to a meeting later that summer and met some awesome women!

The first time I went to church following surgery was Easter Sunday. It was a very emotional day for me. I think I cried from the time I got there until I left, and the tears steadily flowed as we sang the hymn "Because He Lives":

> Because He lives, I can face tomorrow.
> Because He lives, all fear is gone.
> Because I know He holds the future…

I knew with God, I could face this and get through it.

On April 6th, I went for my Positron Emission Tomography (PET) scan. I prayed during the whole scan that there was no more cancer anywhere in my body. Thank the Lord, the PET scan showed no cancer!

I had my port put in on April 8th. The next day I had a Multiple-Gated Acquisition (MUGA) scan of my heart to be used as a baseline, because some types of chemotherapy drugs may damage the heart. That night I went and got my hair cut shorter.

I knew my hair would be coming out and I wanted it to be short so it wouldn't be so drastic (if that was possible).

On April 13th, my husband Randy took me for my first chemo treatment. My nurse that day explained everything she did and told me about each drug that I would be getting. I was given Cytoxan, Taxotere, and Adriamycin. She told me that most people call the Adriamycin the "red devil." She said she had a patient once who refused to call it that and instead called it "the blood of Jesus Christ." That is what I chose to call it, too, because Jesus Christ was helping me get through all of this! He was killing any and all cancer in my body.

I also met with a genetics counselor on this day and had the BRCA gene test. The result from this was negative.

The next day I was given a Neulasta shot to boost healthy white blood cells. I would receive a Neulasta shot the day after each chemotherapy treatment and then go for lab work on Mondays between treatments. This would become my routine for six rounds of chemo. I was blessed to have either Randy or my daughter, Rachel, go with me for all my chemotherapy sessions. The week after my chemo treatment I was usually weak and tired and would sleep a lot. I would have a good week, then another treatment.

The week after my very first treatment, I was very dizzy and lightheaded when I got up, so I had to stop taking my blood pressure medicine. The chemo also made me go into menopause. Yay for hot flashes – NOT!

About two weeks after my first chemo treatment, my head was very tender and sensitive and my hair started coming out, so

I had my husband and daughter shave my head. I know that really bothers a lot of people, but surprisingly, it did not bother me as much as I thought it would. I remember looking in the mirror for the first time and I saw my brother Farrell looking back at me! I had never realized how much we favored one another.

I had a great support system and a lot of people praying for me throughout my diagnosis, surgeries, and treatments. They included my husband, daughter, mother, mother-in law, father-in-law, two brothers, sister-in-law, nieces, nephews, other family members, friends, church family, support groups such as The Rack Pack, and the Lawrence County Breast Cancer Group, and I can't leave out my two dogs who were great therapy. There are too many to name them all. (I know I would definitely leave someone out, too.)

Farrell, my oldest brother, is such an inspiration to me. He was diabetic, on dialysis three days a week, had both legs amputated because of the diabetes, and still had the greatest attitude of anyone I have ever known. He always had a smile on his face when others were around and always asked how you were when you knew he wasn't feeling well himself. He recently passed away, but I will always remember his wonderful attitude.

One of my cousins, Cornelia Hutto, sent me an encouraging, handwritten letter every week and included Scriptures, quotes, and jokes. I found myself looking forward to that letter every week. Laughter is great medicine.

The Friday night before my second treatment was Relay for Life. I was blessed to have a team in my honor. Anita Linderman, a friend since childhood, came up with the idea and several other friends and family participated. Some members of my graduating class also took part in it. I was the third member that I know of from our class to be diagnosed with breast cancer. One of those was a man. Yes, men can have breast cancer too! My team sold enough luminaries in my honor to spell out the words LOVE, HOPE, and CURE in the bleachers of the football stadium. It meant so much to me to know they were there to support me.

After my hair came out I attended a Look Good, Feel Better class, which is open to all women with cancer who are undergoing chemotherapy, radiation, or other forms of treatment. There, they show you how to do your makeup, especially your eyebrows. Your eyebrows and eyelashes, along with all hair on your body, comes out just like the hair on your head during chemo. The plus of not having hair was that I didn't have to shave my legs or underarms. Yes! They also demonstrate ways to wear scarves for headcovers, and gave participants a bag full of makeup. I would recommend this to any female going through chemotherapy.

Between my 3rd and 4th treatments, I went to the beach with Randy and Rachel. We had a great time and it was so good to get away from everything for a few days. I was so thankful that God allowed me to feel well enough to go on this trip.

During chemo, food did not taste right. I wanted spicy foods because they had more taste to them. Instead of losing weight during my treatments, I ended up gaining about 30 pounds. Fortunately, I never got sick to my stomach; I think it helped that I would take a Zofran and eat a cracker before getting out of bed in the morning. I did this for 3 or 4 days beginning about the 3rd day after each treatment.

My last chemo treatment was July 27, 2015. I also went to physical therapy on this day for lymphedema in my right arm. The therapist massaged my arm and showed me how to do it. The massaging helped after just a few therapy sessions, and I still massage it occasionally if I notice any tightness in that arm.

My first radiation treatment was on the 27th of August. I had radiation Monday through Friday for 28 treatments. The radiation treatments were so much easier than the chemo. They made me a little tired, but nothing like the chemo! I was vigilant about keeping cream on the radiated areas. They did turn red like a bad sunburn and peeled, but I did not have the blisters like some people. My last radiation treatment was October 6th, and I got to ring the bell!

The surgeon removed my port on November 13th, then a little over two weeks later I had a PET scan and it was clear. Thank the Lord!

One of my doctors told me that ovarian cancer is linked with breast cancer, so on January 26, 2016, I had a hysterectomy.

Finally, after almost a year from my first surgery, I had the second part of my reconstruction surgery on March 1, 2016. My expanders were replaced with saline implants. I only had two drains this time and they were removed about a week later. I was so glad to get the expanders out because they were so hard and uncomfortable. The implants feel better, but they're still uncomfortable to me, especially on my right side where I had radiation. That implant is harder than the one on the left.

In April 2016, I had a follow-up MUGA scan and it showed no damage to my heart. Again, thank you, Lord!

I have learned to enjoy the small, everyday things, even the mundane things. Sometimes when I am cleaning house, I just thank God that I am here and have the opportunity to do it. I want to enjoy life and not put off doing things that I want to do.

Life on earth is short! Enjoy life! Most of all, make the most important decision of your life and accept Jesus Christ as your Savior and you can have everlasting life in heaven with Him!

Chapter 7
Julie McAbee

"Remain in me, as I also remain in you. No branch
can bear fruit by itself; it must remain in the vine.
Neither can you bear fruit unless you remain in me.
I am the vine; you are the branches. If you remain in
me and I in you, you will bear much fruit; apart from
me you can do nothing." — John 15:4-5 (NIV)

Breast cancer officially became part of my personal life story
in December 2015. My life was forever changed with a
phone call three days before Christmas, but when I take time to
reflect back upon prior events I can without a doubt see God's
guidance, hand, and preparation, and the real beginning of my
story four years earlier.

I've taught 1st and 2nd grade for 22 years. It's my calling, my
heart, my mission field. I love all my students, but in the 2011-
2012 school year I grew to dearly love one particular little girl. I
was new to her school and so very excited to be there. She was in
my first-grade class and she was absolutely precious. Her mother

was diagnosed with Stage 3 breast cancer over Christmas break that year, and we were all heartbroken. The girl was determined to be strong and brave at home. She would not let her momma see her cry, but she would come to school, crawl up in my lap, and sob. I would hold her and cry with her day after day as her momma faced a mastectomy and eight rounds of chemotherapy.

I've heard it said that cancer doesn't become real until it has a face. That year cancer became so very real to me. Because of that sweet girl and her momma, we formed a Relay for Life team. We reached out in various ways to encourage cancer patients and survivors, and I met multiple other courageous, strong women who had survived breast cancer. There's no way I could have known it at the time, but God was giving me a team of women who would help me weather my own storm in just a few short years.

Almost four years later I felt that God was telling me to move on to another school. It was something I felt deep in my spirit with great certainty. There are very few times in my life that I've heard God's direction so clearly, so I requested a transfer and doors opened in such a way that I knew it was definitely God's plan to go.

In August 2015, I was getting settled into my new classroom and my new principal asked that I come up with a personal mission statement to be displayed at school. I began to pray and think about what my mission in life was. One morning during my quiet time I read a devotional written by Wendy Blight. This statement penetrated my heart: "I want my life to bear much fruit. Much love. Much grace. Much joy. Much hope. Much wisdom."

I knew that's what I wanted my personal mission to be, not only as a teacher, but also as a Christian, and that became the prayer of my heart.

About a month later I once again heard God speaking to my spirit. He simply said, "Something big is coming." I thought it had to do with my new school and my new mission field there, but I was mistaken. God was about to create an entirely new ministry in my life that could only be born from my own cancer diagnosis.

Because of my experiences with my student and her mom, I was very diligent about getting my mammograms. In August of 2015, I went for a mammogram and was given the great news that everything was fine. I was told, yet again, that I had very dense breast tissue, but there was no real concern.

I was happy and went on with my life until that November. I found a lump in my right breast while taking a shower. I'd found lumps in the past and had even had three lumpectomies in previous years, but somehow deep in my heart I felt this one was different. I was very concerned. I called my doctor and he worked me in as quickly as possible.

After waiting for my biopsy results for a week, I finally received a phone call. I'll never forget his words. "Mrs. McAbee, you have a malignancy. It's slow growing and nonaggressive, but you have a malignancy. Do you understand? Can you stay on the line to make an appointment to come in to our office?"

My world absolutely stopped. I didn't really comprehend the somewhat optimistic words "slow growing and nonaggressive." In my mind I simply heard, "You have cancer, and you're going to die."

My husband wasn't home from work yet when I received my diagnosis, but my 11-year-old son was home with me. I will forever remember going to my walk-in closet, closing the door, and sobbing like never before. I've always heard of getting on your face in prayer before God, but there's nothing like a cancer diagnosis to bring you to that exact place. In time I learned that there was no better place to be, but at that particular moment my world was shattered and I was gripped with an overwhelming fear of the unknown. How far had my cancer spread, and most importantly would I live to see my baby grow up? So many things were out of my hands, and I was utterly terrified.

You see, I am a bit of a control freak. I like very much to have all my ducks in a row and to have my plans in order. I find great comfort in feeling in control, but cancer has taught me the powerful lesson that I am really not in control of anything in this life. I smile now and tell people that's part of the reason God allowed cancer to be a part of my story. He wanted me to see that I am not at all in control, but that I am deeply loved by the One who is.

After telling my husband my biopsy results, I needed help and guidance from someone who truly understood. Remember the little girl's mom with breast cancer from four years ago? She was the second person I told. She literally scooped me up into her arms and walked with me through every single step of my cancer journey. She and the other women God had brought into my life previously became a support group like nothing I'd ever known before. They cried with me and prayed with me. They calmed my fears and strengthened my faith. They answered millions of questions and helped me make very difficult medical decisions. They pointed me in the direction of fabulous doctors, and they were there 24 hours a day to simply love me.

I tell newly diagnosed women that this "pink club" is not one that anyone wants to join, but once you're diagnosed you are loved and surrounded by an amazingly beautiful group of women who will never leave your side.

Christmas that year was anything but ordinary. I found myself in such a strange place emotionally. We decided we didn't want to tell our friends or family anything until we knew more, so we tried to carry on as if nothing were wrong. My time out of school gave me a chance to begin to process my diagnosis.

A survivor sister had encouraged me to be honest with God and to pour out my heart to Him, and that's exactly what I did. I poured out my fears and He began to meet them one by one as they surfaced. Songs, Bible verses, devotions, and quotes took on a whole new meaning as God used them to speak to me. Things that I'd heard over and over now stopped me in my tracks because they penetrated my very soul. Everywhere I turned God was whispering His hope and His strength into my life. It was humbling. I'd never felt so loved.

After waiting for what seemed like an eternity due to the holidays, I was finally able to meet with my doctors to come up with a plan. I chose to have a bilateral mastectomy since my cancer had gone undetected in my mammogram. I wanted to do anything I could do to prevent a recurrence.

Once our plan was in place we knew we needed to tell our friends and family. In the midst of that most difficult time, God reminded me of a church sign I had seen years earlier: God never wastes His children's pain. I held on to that hope, and I began to pray asking God to take this cancer and to turn it into something beautiful.

As I explained my diagnosis to friends and loved ones, I asked them to agree with me in prayer that God would indeed make something beautiful from this cancer. Once again God was faithful. He had a perfect plan in place and He was working to bring it to pass.

In the days before my mastectomy I began to ask my survivor sisters for information that I would need as I recovered. I also began to look on Pinterest for mastectomy tips. The day before my surgery I ran across a very funny shaped pillow that was specifically designed to help after a mastectomy. I found the directions for how to make it and asked my mom if she could please help me. She purchased the needed items and made it that very day. As I recovered from surgery, my pillow was my absolute favorite item. It offered protection and comfort and gave me the ability to get much needed sleep. I continued to use my pillow for weeks after surgery. About six weeks after my surgery I sensed God telling me to make these pillows for other women facing mastectomies. I asked my mom if she would be willing to help sew them, and our pillow ministry was born.

Time passed. I slowly recovered from surgery, began the reconstruction process, and waited for the test results that would decide if I needed chemotherapy or not. We were blessed with an early diagnosis. My lymph nodes were clear with no sign of cancer, but because I was only 44 when I was diagnosed, my oncologist wanted to run genetic tests on my tumor itself.

When the test results were in, we learned that I had a medium risk of recurrence and the decision was made to do four rounds of preventative chemotherapy. It was not what we had hoped for, but I had fervently prayed asking God to do what was best, so we walked forward knowing that God was good and in control. Five months passed from the time of my diagnosis until my final round of chemo, and my final reconstruction surgery was two months afterward.

I am still in awe when I look back and see God's hand so evident in my life. He placed me exactly where I needed to be when I needed to be there. I had the privilege of loving a hurting family as they faced breast cancer, and they in turn loved me fiercely when I was diagnosed. God gave me a heart years ago to minister to cancer survivors, and they loved and blessed me in return. It is a truly beautiful thing to see God's people love one another, and it's an even more beautiful thing to be used by Him to love others.

One of my most favorite verses that reflects that idea is 2 Corinthians 1:4 – "God comes alongside us when we go through hard times, and before you know it, he brings us alongside someone else who is going through hard times so that we can be there for that person just as God was there for us" (MSG).

It has now been 17 months since my breast cancer journey began. The transformation in my faith and my life has been so amazing that I almost don't recognize myself! And that's not just because my once straight hair is now very curly! I have learned

2222

2

that hard times can, do, and will come. I have learned that God is faithful and won't leave us in that hard place forever. He will deliver us in His time and in His way.

Most importantly, I've learned that God never, ever leaves us alone. And, when we have made it through we are left with a gift beyond compare...we have grown to know Him in a way we'd have never known Him otherwise. We've spent time held tightly in His arms and He has carried us near His heart every single step of the journey. I now know beyond a doubt that the next time (and the next time and the next time) a hard thing comes, He will carry me through once again, because that is who our Heavenly Father is. "When you pass through the waters, I will be with you; and through the rivers, they shall not overflow you. When you walk through the fire, you shall not be burned, nor shall the flame scorch you" — Isaiah 43:2 (NKJV).

God has graciously answered my prayers to bear fruit for Him. I have learned that in order to be fruitful we must face hardship as well as times of joy. We must be pressed and broken to become less like ourselves and more like Christ. While cancer wasn't what I wanted or prayed for, God has used it to change me and to give me the desire of my heart.

We have now given away more than fifty pillows to women facing mastectomies. Our ministry has officially become Comfort and Joy Pillows. Our mission is to provide much needed comfort and to remind hurting women that joy can be found in Jesus even during our darkest of times. I include my contact information (just in case they don't have a pink sister and need one), a brief letter telling my story, and my most favorite Bible verse — "Don't panic. I'm with you. There's no need to fear for I'm your God. I'll give you strength. I'll help you. I'll hold you steady, keep a firm grip on you" — Isaiah 41:10 (MSG).

Cancer has taught me that our God is always faithful, always good, and always at work in our lives. He can take even the worst of things and make them beautiful. He never leaves us, and His ways are perfect even when we don't understand. Hold on to Him, my pink sister. He will never let go, and He can be trusted. I promise.

Chapter 8

Courtney McCollum

"Surely your goodness and love will follow me all
the days of my life, and I will dwell in the house
of the Lord forever." — Psalm 23:6 (NIV)

M arch 10, 2009, was the day that forever changed my life.
That was the day that I found out I had breast cancer. It
was heartbreaking, shocking, and devastating. When you hear the
"C" word, you think this is it, like it is a death sentence. You're
so overwhelmed with emotion that you can't think straight and
it's very hard to comprehend what the doctor is trying to tell you.

I need to back track seven months to when I first discovered
my lump. My family and I were at my son's baseball tournament
when I found it. It was late in July and we had been out in the heat
all day. When I got back to the hotel room I took a long shower
and that's when I first noticed the lump on my right breast. I knew
that it felt different from other lumps that I felt from time to time.
It was about the size of a blueberry, unlike some of the small BB-
sized lumps I had felt in the past, which went away on their own.

I decided that I would make an appointment when we returned home from the tournament and see my OB-GYN.

Two weeks later, I went to my appointment with my doctor. He felt it and said he didn't think it was anything to worry about, but he went ahead and ordered a mammogram and ultrasound. I went for my tests and they told me my doctor would be in touch with me in a few days to go over the results.

My doctor called with the results and said it was good news. Nothing abnormal, it was just a cyst. He added that it may change in size and get either larger or smaller. I asked him if I should follow up with a surgeon to have it removed and he told me that if I were his wife he would not have me do anything. At the time I was 37 years old and thought, "I am young, I don't really have anything to worry about." I was training for my first marathon and felt like I was healthy and in great shape.

Fast forward to February and I noticed the cyst had grown from the size of a blueberry to that of a plum. I thought that I really needed to have the lump looked at again. I was due for my yearly exam with my doctor and figured I would have him check it then. The day of my appointment I saw the nurse practitioner because my doctor was out sick that day. After examining the perceived cyst, she told me that it didn't look normal and wanted me to see a surgeon as soon as possible.

I became a little worried since she got me an appointment so quickly with a surgeon. I saw her on a Thursday and my appointment with the surgeon was the next Monday. My husband decided to go with me because I was a little nervous and didn't know what to expect. Well to be honest, I was really nervous!

The surgeon met with us and decided to go ahead and do an ultrasound-guided needle biopsy. I didn't know if this procedure was going to be painful, but the doctor and his nurse told me it should not hurt and only take a few minutes to complete. It turned out to be quite painful, because my tumor was so large and dense. The needle bounced off the tumor, but after several attempts they got the samples they needed. After he finished with the biopsy, he said he would be in touch with me with the results in a few days.

I attempted to go about my life as normal as possible for the next 24 hours and tried hard not to worry. I wasn't working outside of the home at the time so I could focus on raising my two sons, ages 6 and 11. With children this age, staying busy isn't hard to do. I really didn't have time to focus on my worries. My husband and I had just gotten the boys to bed that next night and were sitting down to watch TV when I got the call that changed our lives.

My surgeon said he knew I had young children and wanted to wait until he thought they were in bed before he called to share the results of my biopsy. I knew it could not be good if he was calling me at nine at night. He told me I had invasive ductal carcinoma. I will never forget that feeling of hearing those words, "You have cancer." I was stunned, shocked, and could hardly comprehend what he was telling me. I felt, I am too young to have cancer! I am in good shape and eat the right foods.

We sat down with my doctor the next day to review my options when he told me that with the size of my tumor, I would need a mastectomy. He also informed me that I would have to do chemotherapy and possibly radiation. I am so thankful that my husband was there with me to take notes and ask questions because I was still in shock.

My doctor made me feel like I was his only patient that day. He spent two hours going over what we should expect with my surgeries and treatment. He put things in motion and I was on the fast track to get this cancer out of my body. That night my husband and I sat down with our boys and told them I had cancer. My 6-year-old did not quite understand, but my 11-year-old did. We told them what to expect, that the chemo would make my hair fall out and make me feel bad.

The next week was full of doctor appointments, tests, and more tests. My oncologist thought it was a good idea to have a PET scan and he also wanted me to have another biopsy. This biopsy would be on my lymph nodes under my arm. During his exam he felt a few that seemed to be enlarged. At this point, I was so tired of being poked and stuck with needles I didn't know how I was going to do this for the next 6 months.

This was one of my first breakdowns that I had during this whole journey. I remember sitting in the room waiting for the doctor to come in and breaking down, crying like a baby. My husband just held me and told me it was ok to cry. He was going to be with me every step of the way.

I got the test results from my second biopsy and PET scan. I had cancer in every lymph node that they tested. My doctors scheduled my surgery for March 27th. This was the day I would have this awful cancer removed from my body.

By now my family, friends, and church were reaching out

to me letting me know that they were thinking about me and praying for us. It was hard retelling my story and what was going on repeatedly to those who asked. That's when my husband and I decided that we would start a Caring Bridge page to keep everyone updated. It amazed me how many people read my story. Some people I had never met, others were old classmates and my friends. Their kind words and prayers were what I needed. I felt so much love and could feel their prayers wrapping around me like a warm blanket.

I was ready to get started with the plan that my doctors had mapped out for me. It was going to be a long process of surgeries, chemo, radiation, and more surgeries. I didn't have a choice; I had to fight. I wanted to see my children grow up, and I wanted to be able to grow old with my husband. On March 27th, I underwent a bilateral mastectomy without reconstruction. I knew that I was in God's hands when my surgeon prayed for me before the operation started. His demeanor and attitude was that God was the Healer, and he was just His tool.

They were unable to do the reconstruction because I had so many lymph nodes that tested positive for cancer. My cancer was stage 3C, one small step away from stage 4. I was on the road to recovery from my surgery and had to heal for a month before I started my chemo.

Through this whole process, I wanted to keep my life as normal as possible. I did not want to think of myself as sick. I wanted to keep going, doing the things I loved — being a wife and a mom.

Both my boys were playing baseball during that particular

spring and a large part of my and my husband's friends were other parents of our boys' ball teams. Several of my close friends organized a surprise for me at the ball park. Moms and kids wore "I Love Courtney" shirts they had made to show support, and that they were there for me for the long battle ahead.

I was finally able to start my chemo in May. The first round was pretty rough and was a shock to my system. I was in really good shape from running and training and I wanted to continue to run during my treatments. Running had always been my "me" time. I found it therapeutic being outside and pushing my body to its limits. But running during my treatments started a different relationship with God. I was not raised in the church. We were that family that attended Christmas and Easter. It wasn't until I got married that I really started attending church and getting involved.

My relationship with God changed after I started my treatments. When I went for runs, I found myself talking with Him. I was able to share my fears, concerns, and dreams with Him. My "me" time turned into the best part of my day. I would cry, scream, and laugh through my runs. It was the first time in my life that I really felt at peace. Even though I did not know what was going to happen to me, I had faith that He was going to see me through this journey. He was going to be there for me and I could count on Him.

Toward the end of my treatments, my body and mind were worn down. Some days I would cry and have short pity parties for myself. I felt like I needed to do this so I could move forward and heal. I allowed myself to do this as long as I got it out of my system and put my big girl panties back on and continued to fight.

The 7th round of chemo was probably the worst. It was the day after treatment and no one was home at the time. I felt so bad and started praying to God asking Him to please help me get through this. I was bald; I looked and felt like death. At that moment, for the first time in my life, I felt God's presence. It was this wonderful sensation of being held and I was overwhelmed with this sense of peace. I was tired and down, but I had Him with me.

This past spring, I celebrated my 8th year "cancerversary." My husband suggested that would be what we call the cancer-free anniversary. He has been my rock though it all. He kept me focused and always told me, "One step at a time, one day at a time. Don't get ahead of yourself and don't think 'what if.'" I would not be where I am today without him and my family. They are what I live for.

Breast cancer was a gift from God. I really didn't want the gift. I didn't like unwrapping it and finding all the ugly surprises in store for me, but it was a gift all the same. I have become much closer to God because of it. I have been able to share my story and build relationships with other women fighting this battle. I would have been too shy before the gift to ever step out like this. Now I talk with total strangers about this disease and offer them support and a shoulder to lean on.

We truly don't always know His plan for our lives. We may never understand His ways, but still, God has a plan for us. Walking in faith, only one step at a time, He led me to the still waters and green pastures of Psalm 23: "Surely his goodness and love will follow me the rest of my days and I will dwell in his house forever." (NIV)

Chapter 9

Cindy Meadows

"I can do all things through Christ who strengthens
me." — Philippians 4:13 (NKJV)

Philippians 4:13 is a verse I had heard quoted many times.
It's a verse I had faith in. "I can do all things through Him
who strengthens me." I knew I would succeed at anything, with
God on my side, but I had never really been challenged. That all
changed on March 5, 2012. It was a day that put a fear in me so
great my faith would be shaken and the source of my strength
eventually revealed.

"It's cancer." I'll never forget those words. A fear swept over
me. Cancer was something I had never thought of having before.
No one in my family had ever had cancer. I was healthy. How
did I get breast cancer?

The initial shock was almost too much to handle. I could
hardly breathe. What would I tell my three precious boys, who
were 11, 13, and 15 at the time? I couldn't die and leave them
so young! How sick would I become? How would I break such

painful news to my mom and dad? How would my husband Barry and I cope with this? Breathing was difficult.

I hung up the phone. We got our boys to bed, pretending everything was okay. I collapsed afterward in Barry's arms, wondering how we would get through this. All I could think about was how I could never leave my boys. I had to see them grow up. I had to see what wonderful things they would accomplish in life. My heart was racing. My stomach was weak. I was scared to death. Within minutes, I called my sisters, planning to go to my parents the following morning just before an appointment with the surgeon. Somehow, we fell asleep during the night. We were exhausted, in shock, and terrified.

The following morning I was numb. I went through the motions of getting my boys to school. Telling my parents was one of the most difficult things I had to do. They were both so shocked and heartbroken. They both cried in each other's arms. My heart ached so badly to have to put them through this, but my mom almost immediately said, "Well, what's our next step?" Those simple words from my mom gave me all the strength I needed to push through the day.

The day was difficult and surreal. We told our entire family, including our boys. Their responses were so innocent. William, a high school sophomore, wanted to be sure that we did not hide anything from him. We promised we would not; of course, we also knew we would not tell them anything they didn't question. Thomas, an 8th grader, wanted to be reassured I was not going to die. Davis, a 6th grader, wanted to be sure he could still play baseball that season.

It made my heart happy to see that they thought of themselves, just as children do. Even though my insides were torn up, I held it together for them. We wanted to do everything possible so they would not to be afraid or worry about me or what would happen to them. Our main goal with the boys was to have normalcy.

My mom planned to stay with us, so Barry, my sons, and my sisters could keep life as normal as possible. We told our boys that cancer would not define us as a family, but the way we fought it would.

Within days of my diagnosis, my sisters had all the family over to our house for dinner and an evening of laughing, playing, and lots of conversation. Our house was full of happiness. My family knew me well. They knew that there was nothing I loved more than being in the middle of all of them. Their love gave me strength to battle through the toughest fight of my life.

Throughout my journey my family was right by my side. Being raised in a Christian home, our family naturally prayed diligently about my diagnosis and upcoming surgery.

The outpouring of love to our family was also very humbling. One afternoon several cars pulled up in front of my house. Teachers from the school where I taught fourth grade started piling into my garage with boxes of paper products and drinks. Others filled our deep freezer with casseroles, desserts, and other frozen meals. My mom and I were speechless. How did they get all this together? They explained that co-workers from my grade level had organized it. Their kindness and generosity gave me strength to face the future.

One morning I let worry overcome me. I was afraid of the

unknown. I decided to call a lady that I knew of from the ballfields who was diagnosed a few years earlier. I had watched her many times and admired her courage. Even though I had my family, I needed to talk with someone who knew how I felt. Courtney and I talked for hours that day. I confided in her, and she spoke to me with honesty. Her words were such a comfort to me, and that day was the beginning of a relationship that would give me strength to not only beat cancer, but later give strength to others.

For the next two weeks, my church family, co-workers, and friends rallied behind us, literally cheering me on to beat the terrible beast of cancer. My faculty and student body held a balloon release and a Relay for Life team in my honor. It was amazing! Hundreds of cards, notes, and Scripture covered a wall in our kitchen, a thick binder, and several baskets.

Our friends from church planned a getaway for us. We spent the weekend in fellowship, song, and prayer. Weeks later they surprised us with a beautiful hammock hanging in our backyard. Meals were delivered to our family for months! All of these acts of love from others gave me strength and hope to fight and win.

It was my OB-GYN who detected the lump in my left breast during an annual exam. Thankfully, he found it and insisted on a biopsy because the cancer didn't show up on the mammogram or ultrasound. I had many decisions to make, but I made them quickly. I was anxious to rid my body of the cancer.

My surgeon advised me to have a double mastectomy, considering my cancer's stealth-like nature. I would lose both breasts. The night before my surgery all three of the boys went to bed with ease. I was so relieved that they seemed worry free, like it was just like any other night. This brought such joy to my soul! That night Barry and I prayed. We prayed most of the night.

Two weeks after my diagnosis I underwent a double mastectomy and the first part of my reconstruction. My surgeon said he could find my family by looking for the crowd. The waiting room was full. The halls were crowded. Dozens of people came to support my family and pray for me during the six-hour surgery and the days that followed.

My mom told me later that a couple of ladies from our congregation brought sandwiches and a cooler of drinks for all of our family at lunch while they waited. This was such a blessing!

When I awoke from the surgery, of course, all of my family was surrounding my bed. There was a very heavy pressure on my chest. Breathing was difficult. They repeatedly told me that there was no involvement in the lymph nodes. The cancer was confined to the breast. There were many tears of joy from everyone, but all I could think about was that my breasts were gone. What did I look like? I was scared.

The unwrapping of my scars revealed me without breasts and with permanent scars to remind me until the day that I die that I had had breast cancer. Barry saw me before I did, and in his typical manner, he immediately assured me that everything was fine. He was overjoyed that the cancer was gone. I'll never forget him whispering to me that he'd never loved me as much as he did at that very moment. His love and commitment to me gave me great strength and courage to look to the future with hope.

Because of my relatively young age and Oncotype DX test results, it was determined that I would benefit from chemotherapy, despite the fact that my lymph nodes were clear. My chemotherapy started four weeks after the surgery. It was brutal. My oncologist said she would fight it aggressively. I would do whatever it took to have the opportunity to raise my boys and grow old with Barry. I was extremely sick throughout the four months of chemo. My mom lived with us most of that time, nursing me every day. She kept going day after day, selflessly giving her all to me.

I got out of the house on any days that I felt up to it and tried to attend church services as much as possible; but I was so sick. I suffered from nausea, weakness, and horrible pain. Pain medication resulted in other problems. My appetite was gone, and I developed sores in my mouth and had severe neuropathy in my hands and feet. I suffered from headaches every day, and my vision was weak. My blood counts were extremely low. There wasn't much that my chemo did not negatively affect. It was overwhelming, but every time I felt like I could not push through to a new day, someone would give me encouragement.

Losing my hair was terrifying. I strongly disagree with anyone who says, "it's just hair." It's much more than hair. My hair was my personality, expressions, and security. Barry and I buzzed it off after I started chemo. After my second treatment, it started falling out. I was terribly sick that day. I remember my sister helping me get in the shower to wash away all the tiny hairs. My scalp was throbbing. I was so weak I could barely hold my head up. The nausea was horrible, but I believed God was going to get me through this. He was carrying me every step of the way.

Throughout my sickness, Barry remained steady. For months I cried every time we were alone. I was overwhelmed with guilt and depression. I wanted desperately to go back in time, but he would always say he would never go back. He was relieved the cancer was gone. He continually told me this and showed me love until finally I quit crying when we were together. The tears vanished as I started focusing on how blessed I was to have a man like Barry, who had adhered to our wedding vows, and loved me in sickness and in health for over twenty years.

I remember lying in my bed one night thinking I felt like I was dying and could not push through another day. That's when I heard my boys in the den talking and laughing. Their laughs were priceless. My heart filled with joy. I cried because I was so happy that they were happy and living life to the fullest. The strength I gained through my boys carried me through four horrific months of aggressive chemotherapy. At my weakest moments, their presence gave me strength to beat the beast.

My friendship with Courtney grew. In the spring of 2013, we decided to start a support group for local breast cancer survivors. The Rack Pack began meeting once a month for dinner. Our mission was to give support to local ladies diagnosed with breast cancer. It's vital to us to make a difference and to give back. Being a part of this wonderful group of survivors and experiencing the results in our community gave me strength to continue my own journey, even after the initial fear of cancer had faded.

As time has passed, I've experienced many emotions concerning having breast cancer and the permanent results from it. They are visible. They are humbling. No matter how much cancer has altered me, Barry remains constant. He loves me unconditionally. Our marriage has only strengthened. We appreciate things we took for granted before. Cancer slowed us down. It gave us wisdom and experiences that made us better people.

Looking back over the last 5 years, cancer has been a blessing. Our boys have experienced life lessons, which have given them courage and maturity. Cancer is tough, but with God we are tougher. I learned that I am strong but only because of who I love. I love God and Christ. I love Barry, my soul mate, my love, my rock. I love my boys, the ones who I adore more than anyone in the world. They are the ones who I live for. I love my family, the ones who have seen me at my lowest and cared for me unconditionally. I love my church family, my friends, and my doctors. I love my mom and dad, who no matter how tired they were, did not give up on me for one second.

When these people gave me comfort or encouragement or love, I was filled with strength from God to do anything…to do all things.

Chapter 10

Dean Norfleet

"God is our refuge and strength, an ever-present help in trouble. Therefore we will not fear..." — Psalm 46:1-2a (KJV)

It was my 43rd birthday, November 18, 1982, the most memorable birthday of my life, which turned out to be the beginning of a new life for me. New in that it caused me to reestablish the priorities in my life and to appreciate my family and friends to a greater degree.

The ordeal began in mid-September when I made a visit to my family doctor at a time that was not the normal time for my annual physical. Even though I had three major surgeries during the previous twelve years, I was not really a "sickly" person, but instead I was an unusually healthy person. I rarely darkened the door of my doctor's office unless I had a real problem, but this time was different. For the past month, I had gone through some extremely stressful family situations causing me to have a different feeling that I had never had before. It wasn't something that put me to bed, nor did it interfere with my job as school teacher, but

I just felt like something was wrong that needed my doctor's attention.

During the normal examination, no obvious problems were found but just prior to my departure from the room, my doctor told me to lie back down on the table so he could examine my breasts, since he had not done that in quite a while. During this examination, he felt a small pea-size lump in my right breast and then made an appointment for me to have a mammogram.

The mammogram a few days later confirmed the lump in my breast, so the next step was to see a surgeon. By that time, it was the first of October and the surgeon's plan was to wait about a month, then check it again and possibly perform a biopsy.

In the meantime, I wanted a second opinion so I made an appointment with a surgeon in a nearby city. The surgeon examined me and my mammogram results and agreed with my hometown surgeon to keep a watch on this, then possibly a biopsy.

During the first week of November, my surgeon, after examining me again, scheduled for me to have a surgical biopsy at our local hospital on November 17th.

From the time of my first doctor's visit in mid-September until the middle of November, I honestly never worried about this problem. I wasn't really a worrier anyway and since no one in my family had ever had cancer, I just didn't give it much thought. I knew I was doing everything I could and should do by seeing the doctors and having the tests and I knew that God was in control, so I just let Him handle it.

My husband and only a very few of my closest friends were aware of the situation at this time. I didn't want the whole world to know it just yet, and especially didn't want our three children to know anything about it. After all, it was only a suspicion and not anything definite and I didn't want all of them getting upset and worried over "nothing." Our children, all in their early 20's, were all away from home, serving in the military — one son in the Air Force stationed in Nevada, one son in the Marines stationed in North Carolina — and both were single. Our oldest, a pregnant daughter, was in Germany with her Army husband and her four-year-old son. Knowing it would be necessary for her to have a C-section to deliver her baby and being halfway across the world, I certainly did not want her to be burdened with worrying about me. Her baby boy was born on Halloween, a month earlier than expected, so she was home from the hospital and recuperating when she learned about my problem.

November 17th came and I had my surgical biopsy. After being awakened in the recovery room, my surgeon had to tell me the bad news that it was malignant. At that moment, I was shocked to hear that news because I had never actually thought that it would happen to me. I immediately had a very serious, heartfelt talk with God. I had always had a close prayerful relationship with God throughout my adult life, but this time it was different. It was like He was right there with me. I told Him if He was ready for me now, I'm ready to go, but if He allowed me to live, I would make each day count in a positive manner and would make it a point to live the rest of my life doing for others and making people happy.

After going from the recovery room to my hospital room, the surgeon came to talk to my husband and me about my options... lumpectomy or mastectomy, which would be done the next day,

November 18th, which happened to be my 43rd birthday. I chose the mastectomy because I did not want to take any chance of cancer cells being missed or reoccurring.

Word about my surgery spread immediately among my family and friends and we then let our children know what was going on. I very quickly began receiving phone calls, visits, cards, and flowers. My hospital room soon looked like a florist, after receiving 42 arrangements of flowers, potted plants, fresh flowers, bud vases, pillow corsages, etc. I had calls, cards, and/or visits from all my siblings and all sixteen of my nieces and nephews.

A few days after surgery, we received the information from the pathology report that even though the removed tumor was malignant, all the lymph nodes that were tested were benign. That was wonderful news to learn that the cancer cells had not spread throughout my body.

I spent twelve days in the hospital, which was a little longer than usual, but there wasn't anything seriously wrong. I just had a low-grade fever a couple of days and for some unknown reason had to have two units of blood. During those twelve days was Thanksgiving, so we got to enjoy a delicious Thanksgiving hospital dinner in my room with my sister and brother-in-law celebrating with us. I was dismissed from the hospital on the Sunday after Thanksgiving and celebrated with another Thanksgiving meal at my sister's house with one of my brothers and sister-in-law attending.

My next doctor's visit was with the oncologist who happened to be new in our city, so I was one of his first patients. Even though no cancer cells showed up in the lymph node pathology report, the oncologist gave us statistics regarding chemotherapy for breast cancer patients and after hearing that, I made the decision to have six months of chemotherapy as a precautionary measure.

I had my first chemo treatment on Friday, the 17th of December, two days before having a celebration on Sunday, the 19th, to celebrate our 25th wedding anniversary, which was taking place the next day on December the 20th. I was a little bit weak for a few days after having the chemo treatment, but did not have any nausea or vomiting that I had previously been warned about so I thought, "That wasn't so bad after all."

I returned to my teaching job the first of January and continued my chemo treatments, having one every four weeks. Even though my first one was without nausea and vomiting, it wasn't the same with my next five treatments. I took each treatment after school on Fridays, via slow drip IV, which took about two to three hours each time. Most of the time I didn't get sick until after arriving home following my treatment, but I would then be VERY sick with nausea and vomiting until Sunday morning, leaving me very weak each time.

I usually lost about five pounds every weekend following a treatment, but would gain it back the next week when I started eating again. Even though I was always still weak on Monday mornings, I was always able to go to work except one time. On Mondays, when I returned to work following my treatment, my wonderful, caring, fellow teachers took turns taking my class to lunch or keeping my study hall class, during their planning periods, allowing me to go to the principal's office or to the teachers' lounge to lie down and rest for about 45 minutes or an hour. How I appreciated the love and kindness shown to me by my co-workers!

During this time of chemo treatments and my terrible times of nausea and vomiting, I tried everything anyone suggested to me to try to prevent those side effects. One of the things the doctor suggested was injections to be taken every 8 hours, first given at the doctor's office just after the treatment, then the next one about 2 o'clock the next morning. Two of my dearest, closest friends who were both RN's, took turns coming to my house at 2 a.m., on Saturdays after the treatments to give me the shots. One lived in a town about 8 miles away and the other lived in a town about 15 miles away, but they both willingly volunteered to provide this service for me. That's really a friend, isn't it? I'm so fortunate to have friends like that.

I was glad when the treatments were over in May. I had been told prior to the chemo that I would probably lose my hair and I thought seriously about getting a wig before I started the treatments but for some reason, decided not to do so. I was later glad that I didn't make that purchase because I lost very little hair and there was no need for a wig. I had very thick hair to begin with and "only my hairdresser knew for sure" about my hair loss.

I continued to get mammograms every six months for about three years, and then annually. Following my surgery, I considered (only for a moment) about having breast reconstruction, but quickly decided that it was not for me. I had no problem with being without one breast, but knowing that if I ever changed my mind I could have it done any time and at any age. Now, nearly 35 years later, I still have no problem with it.

About two years after becoming cancer free, I became a volunteer in the Reach to Recovery Program of the American Cancer Society. The volunteer who visited with my sisters and my husband during my surgery and who visited with me the next day was such a great help to all of us and was a great inspiration to me. With appreciation for her and her interest and kindness, I wanted to be able to provide the same service to other breast cancer patients. I remained in the Reach to Recovery Program for 20 years, then decided to give it up to some younger survivors. During the 20 years of my service, I made visits to hundreds of patients with the intent of providing them with information, hope, and inspiration; however, many times they were more of an inspiration and blessing to me.

I had such great support from my wonderful husband throughout all of this with his love, caring, tenderness, compassion, and help. I also got support in every way from my friends and family and never felt the need to attend therapy sessions offered by Mental Health. I've been so blessed by God placing all these people in my life, helping me to get along so well in every way — physically, mentally, emotionally, and spiritually — as I traveled through the tough times.

I've always known that God, as He promised, would be with me every step of the way and He would protect me during the storms. I have found that to be so very true and am very thankful to have been given the additional years of life after November 18, 1982.

Now, on a lighter note, I must tell you a few of the more humorous things that occurred during this ordeal.

My older sister stayed with me at the hospital the first night after surgery. The next morning I got up to stand at the sink to wash my face and brush my teeth. My sister, sitting in a chair nearby, was carefully watching me as I stood in front of the mirror above the sink, with my right arm close to my chest and my left hand at my waist, pressing my gown close to my body. I said, "Well, when you don't have much to begin with, then you don't have much to lose." My sister, as told to me several times afterward, breathed a sigh of relief when she heard me say that, knowing that I was okay emotionally.

My mode of dress never changed much after this since I was never very physically endowed, I never wore tight sweaters or plunging necklines anyway. It wasn't very difficult getting used to wearing an extra piece of clothing (my prosthesis). I only forgot it one time. I was on my way to school one morning when almost at my destination, I realized I had left it at home. Returning home to get it would have caused me to be late to work, so I just went ahead without it, spent the day at school, and I don't think anyone ever noticed that something was missing.

Another funny thing that happened was the night about three years later as I was getting ready to go to bed, I had placed my prosthesis on the dresser. A few minutes later, my three-year-old grandson who was visiting, came into the bedroom, picked up my prosthesis, and asked, "Grandma, what is this?"

I replied, "That is my boob."

Moments later, after examining it carefully, then placing it back on the dresser, he said, "Grandma, you sure do have a pretty boob!" That was almost 32 years ago, and to this day he has never said another word about my pretty boob.

During the years of these experiences, we attended a small country church in our community. Every Sunday morning at the designated time, those who had a birthday the previous week went to the front of the church and put their pennies in the collection plate — a penny for every year of life — while the congregation sang "Happy Birthday." After my surgery, and having a feeling of "a new life," I put in 43 pennies and $1 for each year thereafter.

One year I was asked by someone why I put in the dollars since they were aware that I certainly wasn't that old, so I told them that "some birthdays are much more valuable than others."

It has now been nearly 35 years since that memorable November 18th, 1982, birthday and I still consider that day to be the beginning of a new life for me, where each day and year is more valuable than the previous ones.

God is so good and I'm so grateful to Him for all He has done for me.

Chapter 11

Kim Tisor

"...do not be grieved, for the joy of the LORD is your strength." — Nehemiah 8:10b (RSV)

I wasn't going to get cancer. After all, it didn't run in my family, I ate fairly healthy and worked out occasionally, you know, when swimsuit season approached. I even had antioxidant-rich green tea in the back of my cupboard...somewhere...in case I got a wild hair to replace my morning cup of cream-laden coffee with it. I didn't plan to hear the "C" word for a long time, if ever. Then again, I didn't plan on gaining the college freshman 15, or allowing my children to watch TV or eat birthday cake before they reached double digits. Life has a way of unfolding in unexpected ways.

It was the middle of July, 2016, when I decided to do a breast self-examination while in the shower. For your knowledge, I checked myself with the same regularity as I attended the gym — when the mood struck. This day I chose to do it and I struck gold, if you can equate finding a cancerous nodule in my left breast to unearthing a hunk of precious metal. Of course, I didn't yet know it was cancer with the certainty found only in the medical community following exams, scans, and biopsies. But, I had a sneaking suspicion.

You would think that my next course of action would have been to make a mammogram appointment, right? Wrong. You see, I planned to attend an upcoming weekend retreat centered on Christ's mercy and I didn't want anything to interfere with that, so I pushed the need for further evaluation of this pesky lump I had found out of my mind. I'm not sure that attending the retreat was more important than seeing a doctor, but a message that I'd receive from the Great Physician while there would change my darkening outlook on life and prepare me to face cancer with more peace, less fear, and a dash of humor. I needed this message and I believe it's for you, too.

The hotel room door closed behind me as I left for the first morning of the retreat when I heard what resembled a whisper into my heart, "The joy of the Lord is your strength." I stopped because the words caught me off guard. Then I heard it ever so softly again, "The joy of the Lord is your strength." Hmmm. "That's odd," I thought. I really didn't know what to make of hearing within my spirit this particular Bible verse, so I dismissed the words as readily as I had dismissed the marble-sized knot embedded in my breast tissue.

Subtle messages centering on the need for joy in our walk with Christ kept surfacing that weekend, to the point that I wondered if they were somehow connected to the familiar verse I had "heard" while leaving my hotel room. Strange. I traveled slightly more than 100 miles intending to learn about our Lord's mercy, but instead it was out of His infinite mercy that He lovingly scrapped my plans, replacing them with His own. Of course, if the Lord wanted me to fully understand what He was doing, He was gonna need to be a tad more direct. (I amusingly assume Jesus appreciates a good challenge when vying for our attention. That's when He gets to show off His creativity best.)

The final day of the retreat while sitting on my bed before checkout I felt the urge to read my Bible. Not knowing what to read that morning, I flipped it open and it fell to the first chapter of Nehemiah. It was impressed upon me to start reading, so I did. I read through chapter 1, then chapter 2, then chapters 3 and 4....

It wasn't clear to me what I was getting out of it, if anything, but I instinctively knew I shouldn't stop. I was prompted to read further. It was like that feeling you have when you're driving, unsure if you're headed in the right direction but you think, "You're probably almost there. Go just one more block." Finally, I reached my "destination." My eyes landed on Nehemiah chapter 8, verse 10, where I found in Scripture as if for the very first time, "...the joy of the Lord is your strength." I had no idea that's where that verse was located. I began to weep.

As the tears fell, scales from my eyes fell with them. The Lord was revealing to me that my joy was gone. Gently forced to take a closer look, I realized it had probably vanished years ago. Oddly, I never noticed. Busy days of rearing children, church activities, tending to the home, and working in radio kept my mind and body steadily moving forward through each day while the joy I once possessed and radiated imperceptibly evaporated into thin air. Thankfully, Jesus had plans for me to recapture what was lost just in time for my breast cancer diagnosis. It's what would sustain me. He's good like that.

By the time I went to the doctor to see if what was still lurking in my breast was indeed cancer, it was near the end of October. My kids were dreaming of Halloween candy and mom-approved costumes while I masked the concerns that were mounting in my heart and mind. Three months had passed since I first found the lump. It hadn't shrunk and felt pretty well anchored into place. The characteristics convinced me it wasn't benign. But how bad was it? Would I be around for future holiday gatherings and our children's birthdays? Or was this it? Would my husband and I celebrate more wedding anniversaries together or did I need to place an ad in search of his next wife? (He probably wouldn't want my help in that area, but it seemed only fair that I should have a say. Wink. Wink.) Either way, I felt an abiding peace knowing I could trust my Savior with the outcome. I knew He loved me too much to allow anything but the very best to happen. I am the Lord's beloved and so are you. We are the apple of His eye.

"He shielded him and cared for him; he guarded him as the apple of his eye."— Deuteronomy 32:10b (NIV)

The OB-GYN I saw, after examining what I thought was cancer, thought it was probably fibrocystic tissue and nothing more, but agreed that it would be wise to have a mammogram. I asked him if we could schedule it for that day. He responded with a quizzical look, as if to say, "You've waited 3 months to see me. What's your rush?"

Nonetheless, his nurse got on the phone to see if there was an opening. When she hung up, she said that they were completely booked BUT they had just had a cancellation and if I could arrive in 15 minutes the slot was mine. I told her that appointment was meant for me and that I would be there. Do you think God had His hand in the timing of that? I certainly do.

The mammogram technician was visibly concerned at the completion of my examination. Worry was written on her face, in her voice, and in her choice of words. Knowing someone in her position isn't to divulge when they've detected some abnormality, I deduced she wouldn't survive in a single round of Texas Hold'em. She informed me to have a seat and wait because I'd probably need an immediate ultrasound. Which I did. As I left for my next appointment, she offered me a free bottle of OPI nail polish in honor of Breast Cancer Awareness Month. I laughed to myself, thinking I probably had breast cancer, but doggone it, this pink, confetti-like nail shellac named "Let's Do Anything We Want" was going to make facing whatever lay ahead all worth it. I do like painted nails.

Several days passed before the doctor called to tell me something suspicious showed up on my mammogram and ultrasound and that I would need a biopsy. When I met with the recommended surgeon, his thoughts aligned with those of the doctor, that what we were dealing with was fibrocystic tissue. OK, I conceded. Maybe I was wrong. Perhaps I had needlessly convinced myself over several months that I had cancer. Even during the image-guided biopsy, as he watched the needle on the screen, the surgeon suggested that it appeared to be a fibroadenoma, basically a benign growth. But alas, what a difference 24 hours can make.

The call came the next morning when the surgeon declared, "It's cancer." It was Friday, November 4th. He told me to meet with him Monday so we could review our options. I thanked him for not making me wait through the weekend for the results, then hung up the phone.

I had no emotional response. Shouldn't I feel something, I thought? I mean, it wasn't my husband who had just called reminding me to pick up his dry cleaning. I was just told that I have breast cancer. Maybe I wasn't stunned or upset because I felt in my heart from the beginning that the lump I had discovered in July was malignant. Perhaps I was benefitting from the divine peace that surpasses all understanding. Perchance it was a little bit of both.

The options presented to me that Monday, scribbled on a piece of paper while I sat on the exam table in my Bounty-esque paper vest, were: A) Lumpectomy with sentinel nodes removed, followed by radiation; B) Single total mastectomy, with sentinel nodes removed and reconstruction, plus mastopexy (lift) on the unaffected side and; C) Double mastectomy and reconstruction. Options B and C included the possibility of follow-up chemotherapy.

I desperately looked for option D where I learn this is all a joke and I could return to life as I once knew it. But upon further detailed inspection, I couldn't find that option printed anywhere. THIS is when the journey started feeling a little uncomfortable. How was I to make the best decision? I wasn't a doctor nor had I ever played one on television. (I'll confess that I played doctor plenty with a childhood playmate, but then we got caught and that ended that.)

I agonized for more than a week, prayerfully considering the right course of action. Honestly, looking back, my prayers were tear-filled frantic pleas for help rather than confident declarations of trust as I sought the Lord's guidance. I don't think anyone would have blamed me for that, but the joy the Lord wanted me to have wasn't going to well up out of a place of worry, fear, and desperation. But, I hadn't fully understood how I was to experience joy. Yet I knew it was mine to have because God had made that abundantly clear to me. And He's not a liar. And He isn't cruel. He doesn't play games of keep-away with His children, dangling gifts of hope, joy, and peace in front of us only to yank them away when we reach for them. Matthew 7:11 came to mind: "If you, then, though you are evil, know how to give good gifts to your children, how much more will your Father in heaven give good gifts to those who ask him!" (NIV) So I asked Him. More on that in a bit.

After much prayer and research regarding options A, B, and C, I made my decision, then changed my mind as I walked into the surgeon's office. Oddly, before I could tell him what I was thinking, he stated exactly what was on my mind: "I think a single mastectomy would be best for you." Peace flooded my soul.

We scheduled the mastectomy for December 6th, which just happens to be St. Nicholas Day, a day associated with gift-giving in many cultures. And, while I didn't initially view having a mastectomy as a "gift," I soon came to accept it as just that. Removing my left breast was necessary if I wanted to rid my body of cancer. It's what would help save and extend my life, along with my oncologist's decision to place me on Tamoxifen for five years. No chemotherapy was required thanks to my Oncotype DX test results.

So, where and how have I discovered joy? It's a daily treasure hunt, but primarily at the feet of my Teacher, Brother, Savior, and Friend, Jesus. I asked Him to rekindle what was once mine and lost. Many mornings begin with me saying or singing, "This is the day the Lord has made, I will rejoice and be glad in it!" (Psalm 118:24, NKJV). Believe it or not, that simple verse powerfully mitigates negative thoughts as we trust that the Lord has something good planned for each new day. After all, He doesn't make bad days, does He?

A dear friend who braved a prophylactic double mastectomy gave me a daily devotional when she found out about my cancer diagnosis that I recommend to everyone. It's called *Jesus Always, Embracing Joy in His Presence*, by Sarah Young. Reading the short entries and their suggested Bible verses each morning help equip me with joy, reminding me that God is always near and intimately involved in all aspects of my life.

When a fear rears its ugly head, I repeat the words on the Image of Divine Mercy I have hanging in my home's sound booth where I conduct much of my radio work: "Jesus, I Trust in You." We really can trust the One who put the stars into place and knew us before we were born with our diagnosis. And with tough decisions. And with our treatment. And with their unpleasant side effects. And with our emotions. And with our future. And with our family's future. We can trust Him with everything, for He's the Lord of all and is over all which includes your cancer and mine.

I believe setting aside time for prayer so you can pour out your heart to God is crucial to cultivating joy. Yes, we're to pray without ceasing, so popcorn prayers tossed up throughout the day are well and good, but nothing compares to one-on-one time with the Creator of the universe who knows us by name. He is

THE SOURCE of joy. Joy isn't something we can manufacture on our own. It radiates from Him and transforms us as we spend time in His presence.

I can't tell you how many times I got down on my knees in front of our living room couch while home alone and just cried while talking to Jesus. The UGLY CRY involving strands of snot and wads of tissues. I always worried during those tear fests that someone would appear at the door and ask what all the wailing was about. Thankfully, there were no surprise visitors. But boy did I feel cleansed afterward knowing I put all my concerns and fears out there and He knew and heard my heart.

I can't say I've ever been angry with God during this entire ordeal, but I know that's a common reaction. If that's you, let me encourage you to still seek Him. He knows that cancer thwarts our immediate plans and dreams and understands that we can become fearful and angry. Yet in our suffering we can still petition the Lord with our desires.

"We do not make requests of you because we are righteous, but because of your great mercy." — Daniel 9:18 (NIV)

Our God is merciful and He is love; that's why we can boldly approach Him to unleash every hurt and disappointment that we've undesirably accumulated. I trust I'll learn more of His mercy as I continue life's journey, but for this season I'll focus on cultivating joy even in the midst of breast cancer. I pray it becomes contagious...my joy, that is...not the cancer. [Envision smiley face here.]

Chapter 12
Marge Wallace

"Be strong and courageous. Do not fear or be in dread of them,
for it is the LORD your God who goes with you. He will
not leave you or forsake you." — Deuteronomy 31:6 (ESV)

I denied the possibility when I was called back for a second
mammogram. After all, I had dense breast tissue that had led
to a false alarm several years before.

I denied the possibility when the radiologist insisted it was
breast cancer. I wanted to ask this know-it-all if he was so certain,
then why do women need biopsies?

I denied it when I went for my biopsy. He too was convinced
it was malignant without completing the test process. Another
show-off.

When I got a call from my gynecologist the day after the
biopsy, I couldn't deny it anymore. My poor doctor had the awful
job of calling me on a Friday afternoon to tell me I had breast
cancer. He gave me the names of two surgeons in town and told
me to call one right away. No more denial.

I told my husband Roger that evening while sitting on his lap, "Yes, it's cancer, but I'm going to be fine." We had the task of raising two granddaughters at the time, one 16 and the other 13. Our first joint decision after my husband was mentally at ease with my diagnosis was that we would not inform the girls until we had a plan in place. I couldn't tell them I had a disease that could kill me with no answers as to what we were going to do about it. So, we had to get a plan.

This was April 2009, and I had started a new job just six short months earlier. Soon after I knew the results of my biopsy I told my boss. She told me that all she asked was that if it became too difficult for me to work and I needed time off to give her as much notice as I could. Love that woman.

The following Monday, she and an attorney from our building came and stood in front of my desk saying they were doing an intervention. I wanted to laugh because my first thought was that I was just diagnosed with stage 3 breast cancer — I didn't have or need an alcohol or drug problem.

It turned out the attorney had gone through breast cancer treatment herself and wanted to help me. She became my mentor. I remember her saying that chemo was awful, and it was. She told me I could get through it and even work while going through it. That is what I needed to hear and that is what I did.

I am a "cradle Catholic," and my job was at an evangelical Christian radio station in Colorado, KTLF. I was surrounded by believers, both at home and at work. My boss assured me that I could be angry at God, that "He was strong enough to handle it." In my mind, though, God had placed me in a position where I had medical insurance, He'd connected me with a medical team I loved, in a Catholic hospital, with a husband and family who were totally supportive. Why on earth would I be angry at God?

For my treatment plan I chose a lumpectomy, followed by 16 rounds of chemotherapy, then 6 weeks of radiation. I've never really acknowledged myself as having breast cancer, or accepted the disease as mine, but I readily claim that I did all of the necessary treatments. That was a challenging season of life that I could never ignore.

I discovered early on that Roger did better if I was doing ok. So many times I had to "fake it 'til I could make it." We had started replacing carpet with wood flooring on our home's main level before all of this "fun" began. We'd only gotten one room done. It was now my husband's job to finish the floors in three bedrooms, a hallway, and a living room by himself. If I tried to help, he had to spend more time worrying about me than if I just left him alone.

Roger also assumed the responsibilities of cleaning the house, doing the laundry, and keeping us all fed. I didn't have the strength to do any of these things shortly after chemo started. Not only is he the best husband on the planet because he took all of this on without a single complaint, he also sat through every doctor's appointment I had, every round of chemo, and remained by my side every day I required radiation. He was and still is the love of my life and my rock.

My best time to pray was early in the morning, in the shower, while Roger drove the girls to school and I was alone in the house. My initial basic prayer was thanking God that my cancer had been found, that I had such a wonderful medical team treating me, that I would remain able to work and be able to keep my hair once I started chemo. My oncologist had told me I was going to lose my hair, but selfishly I'd decided that since God can do anything, maybe, just maybe I'd keep my hair.

Well, two weeks after my first round of chemo, during that prayer time in that shower clumps of hair began to fall out. I did what every logical Christian does. I told God, "Well, I'm not going to thank You for letting me keep my hair anymore." I'm sure God was laughing at my anger that day.

When Roger got home, I was crying as I told him my hair was falling out. He started crying, too, and lovingly uttered the words, "It's working." Duh, I hadn't even thought of that.

At the end of the week, my co-worker, James, brought his clippers to the office. It was a clear day and so we went outside with a chair and he shaved my head. Then he shaved his own. Should you read this, James, I want you to know that was a gift I'll never forget.

During chemo, I had the best medical team imaginable. The nurses were upbeat and fun when it was appropriate, and caring and completely empathetic when that was what I needed. They loved to tease me about being a lightweight because the Benadryl they gave me to minimize any potential allergic reactions knocked me out every time. But while I was out of it, Roger got to meet so many people that were there on the same schedule as I was on. One couple, who listened to KTLF, once brought peanut butter and jelly with them for us to take to the station during our peanut butter and jelly drive to help those in need.

Chemo is about the most difficult thing I've ever gone through. Over the course of six months I did four rounds of Adriamycin and Cytoxan and twelve rounds of Taxol. I also volunteered for a double blind clinical trial, because it made me feel closer to all the women who'd gone through so much suffering in years past to get my treatment to where it was when I needed it.

I still remember driving to the hospital for the first round of chemo. My husband and I were totally silent. I'm sure he didn't know what to say, while I was afraid if I said anything ("I'm not doing this" came to mind) that I would jump out of a moving car. For at least a year after treatment, we could not travel that route without me shaking and crying. I was told it was a form of PTSD.

I did not know a human being could be so tired and remain standing. I continued to work and I remember that besides treatment days, I only took 1½ days off work. I know it wasn't my strength that allowed me to do this, it was God carrying me through those 10 months.

My oncologist told me that I would have more energy if I could get some exercise. I love walking and we had two dogs who loved the dog park. One Sunday morning we decided that I felt up to doing at least one lap around the park. By the time we finished, one side of my face and my arm were purple. Not burnt, but purple. It didn't hurt, it was just purple. When I went to work, everyone was frightened, assuming that I was in pain. That wasn't the case at all. I was just purple. My clinical trial nurse pointed out that she had told me that the sun would have a stronger effect on me during chemo. I felt like she should have told me I needed to wear a burka outside. I stayed away from the dog park after that.

Another odd side effect was that I lost half of my finger nails. They just began popping off one evening. At first I thought it was the gel nail I had on, but upon looking closer, I saw my nail was gone. A friend and I had been going to get our nails done after every other round of chemo. Now that I didn't have all my nails, that was the end of that treat. Also, the lack of hair meant that my eyes teared all the time and my nose ran, constantly, but the inconveniences were offset by the advantage of not having to shave my legs!

Around the time I was done with the Adriamycin and the Cytoxan and eight rounds of Taxol, I didn't think I could continue. On my appointment date for blood work, I began crying and said I just couldn't do anymore. The nurses called my oncologist into the infusion room and he said I could stop if I did one more round the next day. My husband didn't say a word, but the look on his face told me there was no way I could quit. I had to do everything possible to win this fight. So I did it.

I recall that on the Fourth of July friends invited us over for brunch and a movie later. After the brunch I said I needed a nap before going to the movie. It turned into a 12-hour nap. Needless to say, we missed the movie.

I was so fortunate to be treated in a Catholic hospital. I can remember crosses in every single room I ever entered. I remember nuns walking through the halls asking if I wanted them to pray for me and to pray with me. We all want to go home when bad things are happening, and this was almost the worst thing I could imagine. Yet the hospital served as the best home to have to go to, at least here on earth.

I joined an online support group which sadly has over 300 members — women at different places in their journey with breast cancer. We support one another, share information, and keep spirits up when necessary. I've made some wonderful friends on this site.

Most importantly, I know that God brought me through this ordeal. I saw that I could fight a huge battle and win. My husband proved beyond a shadow of a doubt that he took our marriage vows very seriously, especially the "in sickness and in health" part. Roger, you have no idea how much your love and support have meant to me and always will.

I don't ever want to go through this again, but I would not trade the experience for anything. I have been cancer-free, through the help and love of God, since January 2010.

Acknowledgements

There are so many people who deserve to hear the words "Thank you!" from me that I'm reluctant to list them knowing that I'll inadvertently omit people. But let me attempt to list a few...or a couple dozen...

- To my husband, Randy, for believing that I could actually put together a book when I wasn't so sure myself... thank you.
- To my mom, Sherry Hancock, for traveling the distance, literally, to cook, clean, caravan, comfort...thank you.
- To my dad, Dorris Hancock, for being the kind of man that I know would be here sacrificially loving me if Heaven hadn't taken you so soon...thank you. I look forward to our future reunion so very much.
- To my brother David Hancock and his wife, Sandy, and children Jack and Gracie, for your many prayers. I know God heard and answered each one...thank you.
- To my Aunt Jackie Saturley for the visits and shared excitement in publishing *Joy Is Contagious...Cancer Isn't...* thank you.

- To my sisters-in-law Kym Sjauw and Karen Tisor for the flowers, care packages, texts, and making our girls' trip happen. What memories...thank you.
- To Sue Jones for the St. Benedict bracelet...I should consider removing it at some point...and for helping me see labels in an entirely new light during our girls' trip... thank you.
- To all the women in this book for your Christian testimonies and willingness to write and let me share your beautiful stories...thank you.
- To my surgeon Dr. Hugh Nabers for his unmatched bedside manner and friendly staff...thank you.
- To Dr. Gordon Telepun and the staff at Decatur Plastic Surgery for their ideal mix of professionalism and compassion and making me laugh during most visits... plus turning me into a solar eclipse chick...thank you.
- To Dr. Heather Shah for genuinely caring about her patients and patiently listening to every single founded and unfounded fear of mine regarding Tamoxifen's potential side effects...thank you.
- To Ed and Diana Stucky for editing this book and your years of unwavering friendship and constant stream of encouragement...thank you.
- To my boss Robyn Sedgwick and the rest of the KTLF staff for your many heart-felt prayers and phone calls, and for placing my health before performance...thank you.
- To the KTLF listeners for any and all prayers lifted on my behalf and for the timely cards and emails...thank you.

- To the women at First Baptist Church, Black Forest, Colorado, for assembling and sending "The Blue Box." There was a lot of love in that care package!...thank you.
- To the women at Annunciation of the Lord Catholic Church in Decatur, Alabama, for the lunch and unexpected gifts...I say thank you.
- To Father Ray Remke and Father Charles Merrill for the prayers and for administering the meaningful and effective Sacrament of the Anointing of the Sick...thank you.
- To Sister Teresa Walsh for always asking how I'm doing and sticking around for the answer...thank you.
- To Jim Strelec for the daily pep talks that were sometimes firm when I needed for them to be...thank you.
- To Mary Eve Deason for ensuring Mom wouldn't go hungry when she came to our house, ha ha...thank you.
- To Rachel McCubbin for making "that" call when the Holy Spirit prompted you to...thank you.
- To Susan Seyler for your caring support felt hundreds of miles away through your perfect surprise practical gifts, notes, and Facebook messages...I will always cherish your thoughtfulness...thank you.
- To Becky Oldham and Heather Schlitzkus for forgiving me that I wasn't a better friend when you traveled this road before me...you know I love and miss you both... thank you.
- To Kristen Rabideau for the beautifully hand painted and framed Bible verse that brings joy to my heart every time I see it...thank you.

- To Jennifer McDowell and daughter Nicole for releasing a balloon in honor of me and other breast cancer warriors before your softball game. You've forever touched my heart...thank you.
- To Jennifer Kissner for offering moral support and remaining my friend since elementary school. You are special to me...thank you.
- To Stephanie Weathers for the scrumptious meals, warm visit, and willingness to connect me with your endless list of contacts...thank you.
- To Kam Acupan for the thoughtful meals and listening ear...thank you.
- To Anne Palmer for your many encouraging cards, text messages, and personal words of encouragement...thank you.
- To Jan Gile for the best breast book ever and lovingly crocheted prayer shawl...thank you.
- To Peggy Barber for the box full of button-downs and other welcomed and appreciated items...thank you.
- To the best neighbors around for the meals, messages, and offers to help with the kids...thank you!
- And lastly to YOU the reader for taking the time to absorb the stories found on these pages. It's because of you that I believe the Lord inspired me to assemble this book. Thank you and may God richly bless you and yours.

In Him,
Kim Tisor

NOTES and Questions for Reflection

1) What is my biggest fear?

_____

_____

_____

_____

_____

2) Do I believe God can help me overcome my fear? Why or why not?

_____

_____

_____

_____

_____

3) What Bible verses indicate God is with me?
(Write them out and review them often.)

_____

_____

_____

_____

_____

_____

4) Who has God placed in my life to walk this journey with
me? (Expect this list to grow and change.)

_____

_____

_____

_____

_____

_____

5) What spiritual or even physical activities help me feel
closer to God?

_____

_____

_____

_____

_____

_____